HI PHOENIX

FAVORITE DAY HIKES

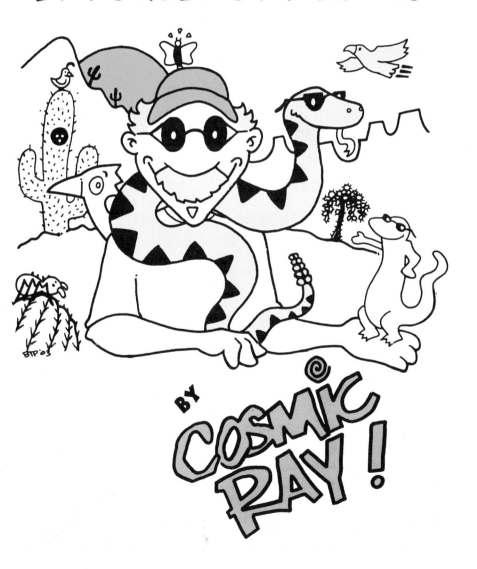

BY COSMIC RAY!

~ CONTENTS ~

BLACK CANYON
BLACK CANYON TRAIL 13

CAMELBACK MOUNTAIN
CHOLLA SUMMIT TRAIL 15
ECHO CANYON SUMMIT TRAIL 17

LOOKOUT MOUNTAIN
SUMMIT TRAIL 19

McDOWELL MOUNTAINS
GATEWAY TRAILS 21
LOST DOG TRAILS 23
NORTH TRAIL LOOP 25
SCENIC TRAIL LOOP 27

NORTH MOUNTAIN
NATIONAL TRAIL LOOP TO SUMMIT 29

PAPAGO PARK
PAPAGO PARK TRAILS 31

PHOENIX MOUNTAINS
CHRISTIANSEN TRAIL #100 33

PICACHO PEAK
SUMMIT TRAILS 35

PINNACLE PEAK
PINNACLE PEAK TRAIL 37

SHAW BUTTE
SHAW BUTTE SUMMIT LOOP 39

SOUTH MOUNTAIN
ALTA/BAJADA LOOP 41
HIDDEN VALLEY LOOP 43
HOLBERT TRAIL..................................45
JAVELINA/BEVERLY CANYON LOOP 47
KIWANIS/RANGER LOOP 49

~ CONTENTS ~

SOUTH MOUNTAIN (CONTINUED)
NATIONAL/MORMON LOOP.................................51
PIMA CANYON TRAILS...............................53

SQUAW (PIESTEWA) PEAK*
CIRCUMFERENCE TRAIL 55
DREAMY DRAW NATURE LOOP 57
MOJAVE TRAIL 59
SQUAW PEAK NATURE LOOP 61
PERL CHARLES TRAIL 63
QUARTZ RIDGE LOOP.............................65
SUMMIT TRAIL.......................................67
*NAME CHANGE TO PIESTEWA IS OFFICIAL, BUT SOME OLD SIGNS REMAIN.
BOTH NAMES ARE TEMPORARILY USED TO AVOID CONFUSION.

SUPERSTITION MOUNTAINS
TREASURE LOOP 69
SIPHON DRAW TRAIL..............................71
HIEROGLYPHIC CANYON TRAIL 73
PERALTA CANYON TRAIL 75
MASSACRE GROUNDS TRAIL 77

USERY MOUNTAINS
CAT PEAKS LOOP 79
MERKL LOOP..81
PASS MOUNTAIN LOOP 83
WIND CAVE TRAIL 85

WHITE TANK MOUNTAINS
BLACK ROCK LOOP.................................87
FORD CANYON TRAIL TO ROCK DAM 89
FORD CANYON/WILLOW SPRING LOOP..............91
WATERFALL TRAIL 93
WILLOW SPRING TRAIL 95

HIGH COUNTRY (SUMMER HIKES)
FLAGSTAFF: HUMPHREYS PEAK TRAIL.................97
FLAGSTAFF: RED MOUNTAIN TRAIL.....................99
PAYSON: HORTON CREEK TRAILS 101
PRESCOTT: GRANITE MOUNTAIN VISTA TRAIL 103
SEDONA: WEST FORK TRAIL 105
SEDONA: WET BEAVER CREEK TRAIL...................107

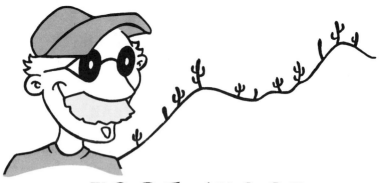

~ FORE WORD ~

In cooking up the recipe for this fun collection of my favorite Phoenix hikes, I have always had before me the rather pleasant-but-daunting challenge of creating a reliable, complete, up-to-date, enlightening and somewhat entertaining guide . . . a tall order with many ingredients. Keep in mind that I am only one guy. I have done all in my power to make this book as clear and accurate as possible, but in spite of my care I have no doubt that there may be a mistake lurking between the pages. Although every hike has indeed been hiked by me, it is at times necessary for me to depend on the words of others . . . others like you. Information has a certain "shelf life". Yes, information does get stale. I earnestly urge any reader who encounters such an error or omission to contact me DIRECTLY via e-mail (cozray@juno.com) and I will quickly pass your correction on to other hikers in future editions. Your help is appreciated. Thank you.

ISBN: 978-1-4951-1993-4
SIXTH EDITION
© 2015 COSMIC RAY

~ RATING THE HIKES ~

For comparison's sake, all hikes were rated by me, a seedy but sincere middle age male in reasonably good physical condition if otherwise unencumbered by any thing even remotely resembling a thought process.

EASY

Flat or possibly some little hills with nothing too steep, too rough or too long. A weenie hike. If you can't handle this you are one hopeless sofa spud. Buy a *TV Guide*. Seek medical attention. Maybe come back later.

MODERATE

Guaranteed to get the dead laughing and singing again. Some interesting terrain with possible combo of minor elements of climbing, a bit of good distance and maybe even some small exposure to risk. Good sweaty, stinky hard work, but still not killer.

DIFFICULT

Some combination of rough, tough, hard, long, steep, rocky and even a possible bit of danger. Not for the weak or respiratorily challenged. Let your most vivid imagination run amok. Sort of like straight espresso. If you don't know what it is, you don't want it. Desert hiking can be unforgiving. Always great to push one's personal envelope, but wise to keep within reason.

SEVERE & EXTREME

Caution! May set off low self esteem panic attack. You may even catch sight of your own blood. All the usual steep, rough, tough, long, thorny, evil nature of a mere difficult hike with a bit of the sick and twisted, self destructive thrown in for good measure. Often hateful and gruesome. Only for those lacking common sense, but sure makes for good stories.

"Some days I feel like there is no reason to get out of bed.
Then I feel wet and realize there is."
- Homer Simpson

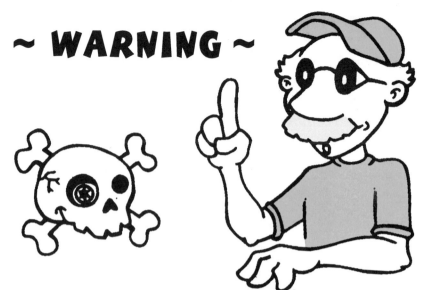

~ WARNING ~

HIKING MAY BE HAZARDOUS TO HEALTH
DESPITE WHAT SOME SLICKER-THAN-A-CHEAP CHICKEN LAWYER MAY WHISPER IN YOUR EAR, IT AIN'T MY FAULT.

THEREFORE: Ray advises that hiking is risky stuff. I have scars to prove it. This book is no substitute for topo maps, route finding skill, compass, good judgement, sense of humor, manners or cognitive thought.

FURTHER: I've done my level best. I'm not responsible for wind, rain, clouds, cacti, snakes, bugs, beasts, boners, rocks, sign changes, puddles, detours or any misfortune that may get your butt fur in a knot.

MOREOVER: Upon buying or otherwise snaking this book and reading this disclaimer you release and discharge me, my heirs, my friends and representatives from mistakes, getting lost or hurt. Hey, awake to the fact that poop happens. Lighten up a little.

REALIZE: It ain't Ray's quackin' fault. It's one's own responsibility to be familiar with route, road, trail, grief factor, weather, water supply, meds, mind set, companions, lions, tigers bears, undies, acts of God, backpack, camelsack and every other dang thing.

FINALLY: It is OK to be weak of physique or lame of brain, but if you be thin of grin, PLEASE STAY SAFE AT HOME! Thank you.

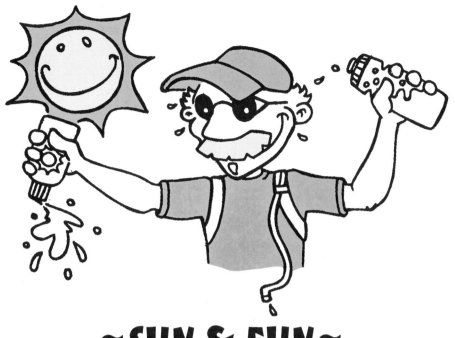

~SUN & FUN~

The sun is either a warm, friendly giant or a relentless, monstrous ogre. Which it will be depends on you. Water is your very best friend. Carry plenty. It may be heavy as you leave the parking lot, but goes away quick as you drink, pour it over your head, soak your shirt, give it away or water the plants. Coffee, tea, beer, pop or even a giant blue slushy from Circle K will not keep you cool and hydrated. They only make you pee and get *de*-hydrated. Your muscles will ache. Your head will spin. You cannot think. You become grumpy and tired. My jokes will not seem funny. Always bring *at least* one to two quarts of water. Carry more as heat, distance and elevation gain increase. A hydration pack that carries your stuff and conveniently delivers water via hose and bite valve is a great idea encouraging frequent sips.

Choose quality UV resistant sunglasses. Bring a scarf for your neck. Wear a hat and light weight, light colored, loose fit clothing. Desert sun feels great on your skin, but a burn may come back to haunt you years down the road. Slather on the high SPF sunscreen. Apply the sunscreen only below your eyes or it will sting like the devil when your sweat causes it to run. Better to wear that hat. Seek shade and avoid hiking when that mid-day summer sun commences to get cranking. From May to September, best to hike only dawn to 10AM or 4PM to dark.

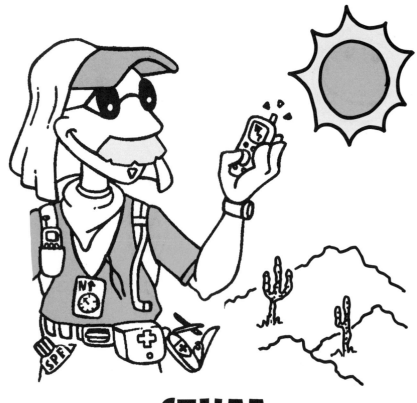

~STUFF~

You are going to need a few items. Here is a suggested list of gear that I've found to be absolutely essential for desert hiking plus a few other optional bits and pieces that may further add to your enjoyment of this fabulous Sonoran Desert. Prior preparation is key to a trouble free experience.

WARM WEATHER CLOTHING

I like to keep the sun off. Wear a nice big hat. A scarf will protect your neck and cools you off when soaked with water. A light colored, loose fitting, long sleeve shirt looks great and keeps your upper body from looking like an alligator by the time you turn 40. Comfortable shorts with ample pockets are great for most hikes. Long pants are best in brush and stickers. Comfortable shoes that have a few miles on them will keep your feet happy. Tevas® are great for creek hikes. Running shoes are fine for short smooth walks. Lightweight walking shoes or boots are good for most of the hikes in this book. Serious leather boots with good support are needed for the serious adventure carrying a heavy load over long distance and rough terrain.

COOL WEATHER CLOTHING

The desert can be cold and wet. Be prepared. Layering is the way to go. In cool or rainy weather I wear a moisture wicking undershirt, a sweatshirt, fleece jacket and a waterproof breathable parka. I can put on a layer or or strip off a layer as the day requires. A warm wooly hat is great to pull down over my ears on a stormy winter mountaintop when a cold wind comes up and the rain and snow begin to blow.

ESSENTIAL GEAR

COMFORTABLE DAY PACK with wide, well padded straps. Not too big. Not too small. Must include pockets for water bottles or allow for a hydration system like a Camelback®.

FIRST AID KIT including moleskin, gauze pads, adhesive tape, band-aids, anti-biotic ointment, alcohol wipes, bug repello and cortisone cream for the itchy bite or thorn. A pocket knife with scissors and tweezers for major or minor surgery. And don't forget the pain killers.

MISCELLANEOUS little stuff like a guide book or map, sunscreen, sunglasses, lip balm, lighter, compass and mini-flashlight for that excellent sunset walk-down-the-mountain-in-pitch-black. Your cell phone is a good idea too, but reception may be iffy in back country canyons. You may want to carry a GPS. (You may be lost, but at least you'll know exactly where you are lost!) However, I doubt you'll need it for any of the well marked hikes in this book. Small, powerful binocs are great for animals, views and close-up birding. Finally, a small camera can capture a single brilliant flower or the memory of a magic sunset when desert glows neon electric for just a few seconds.

FOOD

A short hike under an hour may require nothing but water or little more than a small snack. I prefer an energy bar and maybe a piece of fresh fruit or a few raisins. A longer day hike requires a bit more attention to your energy needs, but no need to overdo it. Stay away from highly processed foods, junk food, candy, candy bars and other fake food. Your engine needs real fuel. If I'm out for a few hours, I like to have good healthy snacks and then at lunchtime, pick out a nice spot with a great view and pull out some fruit and a sandwich made with good bread and other tasty stuff. I might eat it all, I might not. I might save some for later. I never like to feel totally stuffed, especially when I have some good walking to do.

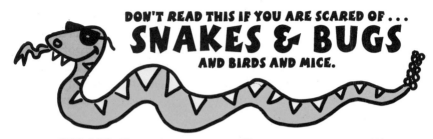

RELAX! Chances are you will not encounter a Western Diamondback Rattlesnake . . . but you might. In any event, they will not attempt to eat you. You are much too large for them to swallow. They want a nice bird, bug or mouse. However, Mr. & Mrs. D. Back Rattler are to be considered armed and dangerous. They will stand their ground and issue warning if you come near. Their buzz is loud and unmistakable. This sound is hot-wired deep in your brainpan. It is meant to make you flee and it works. You will know exactly what to do without giving it a second thought. You will stop dead in your tracks. You will jump straight up and away. Your heart will pound. During your stand off with the snake you will both stare for a few moments and then the snake may or may not yield. If it yields, continue. If not, go way around or go home. This is simply the way it is.

DO NOT attempt to kill, move, poke or prod the snake. Most bites occur when the snake is surprised or when somebody, usually a human male of somewhat less than average intelligence, messes with the snake. Darwin was right, you know.

RATTLERS are like other snakes. They are cold blooded and unable to internally regulate their body temperature. When it is too cold, they sleep. They love to warm up on their trails in their morning sun. When it becomes too hot, they seek shade and move into their cracks and crevices. Look before you grab a hand hold full of sorrow.

DIAMONDBACKS are big, scary things. We name whole baseball teams after them. They usually look just like part of the desert, black and tan plus maybe a little green camo and a diamond pattern on their back. A newborn (live, no eggs) is about 10 inches long. Full size runs, er, uh, slithers about 5-6 feet, although 6 feet would be huge. They have well developed fangs and poison delivery system. They hunt at night and rule the rodent world. Good thing for Phoenix. Their venom attacks the blood system of their prey. They use heat sensitive pits on their heads to "see" their victims even in total darkness. If bitten, your chances of survival are very good, but you must LOOSELY isolate or compress the bite and seek medical attention right away. That's why you pay for a cell phone, silly. DIAL 911.

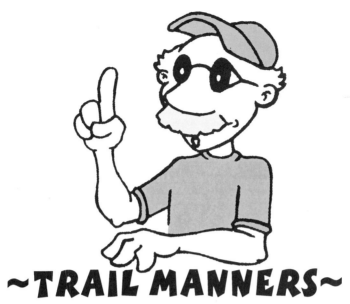

~TRAIL MANNERS~

Death to micro-trash! Leave the desert environment cleaner than you found it so that others may enjoy its natural, pristine, perfect beauty. Butts, matches, peels, cores, crumbs, used TP, wrappers, small bits of found glass, etc. all go in that zip-lock baggie you thoughtfully brought along. Yes, even pack out doggie doodie. Fido is *your* responsibility. Leave NOTHING but your footprints. Do a good deed. Adopt some trash.

Honor the ancient ones who lived here before modern times. Their art is a treasure . . . a direct visible connection to a primordial world of hunters and gatherers going back tens of thousands of years before the dawn of time. Do not touch, rub, fondle or otherwise vandal those petroglyphs and pictographs. Over the years, oils and abrasion from many hands ruin the art. Photograph or enjoy with eyes only. Do not disturb any ruins, either ancient or modern, that you may come across, nor pick up any artifacts. No stealing. You may go to jail and/or acquire a curse. No joke. If you see any such activity, report it to the authorities.

Respect the trails. Your new trail or short cut speeds erosion and kills fragile desert vegetation. A giant saguaro begins life from a seed no bigger than the period at the end of this sentence. Stay on the trail. No fires. No littering. No yelling. No throwing rocks. No shooting. No bad stuff. Just do the right thing and you'll have no problemo. Simply enjoy.

BLACK CANYON TRAIL

©© RAY

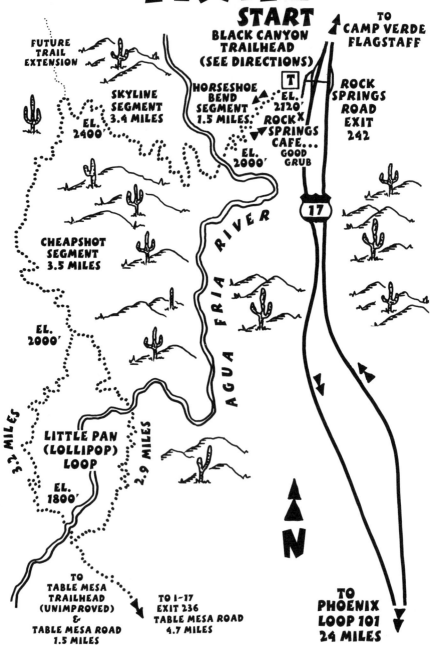

START
BLACK CANYON
TRAILHEAD
(SEE DIRECTIONS)

TO
CAMP VERDE
FLAGSTAFF

FUTURE
TRAIL
EXTENSION

SKYLINE
SEGMENT
3.4 MILES

HORSESHOE
BEND
SEGMENT
1.5 MILES.

T

EL.
2120'

EL.
2400'

ROCK
SPRINGS
ROAD
EXIT
242

ROCK X
SPRINGS
CAFE...
GOOD
GRUB

EL.
2000'

AGUA FRIA RIVER

CHEAPSHOT
SEGMENT
3.5 MILES

17

EL.
2000'

3.2 MILES

LITTLE PAN
(LOLLIPOP)
LOOP

2.9 MILES

EL.
1800'

N

TO
TABLE MESA
TRAILHEAD
(UNIMPROVED)
&
TABLE MESA ROAD
1.5 MILES

TO I-17
EXIT 236
TABLE MESA ROAD
4.7 MILES

TO
PHOENIX
LOOP 101
24 MILES

BLACK CANYON TRAIL
WILD COUNTRY NORTH OF PHOENIX

DISTANCE: 3.0 MI. TOTAL
(A WHOLE LOT MORE IF YOU WANT)

TIME: 2-3 HOURS

EFFORT: MODERATE CLIMB

TYPE: OUT & BACK

ROUTE SKILL: EASY
(TRAILHEAD SIGNED)

BEST SEASON: SEP to JUN
(HIKE VERY EXTRA EARLY IN SUMMER)

PETS: DOGS UNDER CONTROL

AT-A-GLANCE

2600

**ELEV.
(FT.)**

1600

0   **1-WAY MILES**   1.5
(TO AGUA FRIA)

FAVORITE TRAIL

WORTH A JOURNEY

DESCRIPTION: I guarantee this to be a most memorable day hiking through the undulating foothills below the Bradshaw Mountains north of Phoenix. It's a short (but not totally easy) up, over and down to the Agua Fria River for a moderate three mile hike. If the Agua Freddy is not running big, you can check out the map and continue on further. . . even taking a couple of days for a long 23 mile backpack loop. It's gorgeous rolling country. You'll spot nearly every manner of Sonoran cactus, wildflower and wildlife. There are no crowds or anybody for that matter. You'll most likely not see a soul. I came across a desert tortoise out for its morning stroll right in the middle of the trail. I observed from a distance and he showed no alarm. Control your dog in such an encounter.
DO NOT attempt to ford the Agua Fria if running big or flashing. It has quite a push to it and you could easily drown.

Great victuals, especially home made yummy-licious pies, at historic Rock Springs Cafe, just a long stone's throw from the trailhead. Nothing like coffee, pie and ice cream after working up an appetite. And they have real food too.

DIRECTIONS: Take I-17 North out of Phoenix heading toward Flagstaff. Continue 24 miles north of the Loop 101 to the I-17 Rock Springs exit #242. Turn LEFT (West) over the freeway to the stop sign. Turn RIGHT (North) onto the frontage road. Continue about 300 feet to the first road on the LEFT, Warner Road. Turn LEFT onto Warner. Drive to the first crossroad and turn RIGHT to the trail head parking area. As far as I know this parking lot is safe, but best to observe normal caution and stash your valuables anyway.

CAMELBACK
CHOLLA (SUMMIT) TRAIL

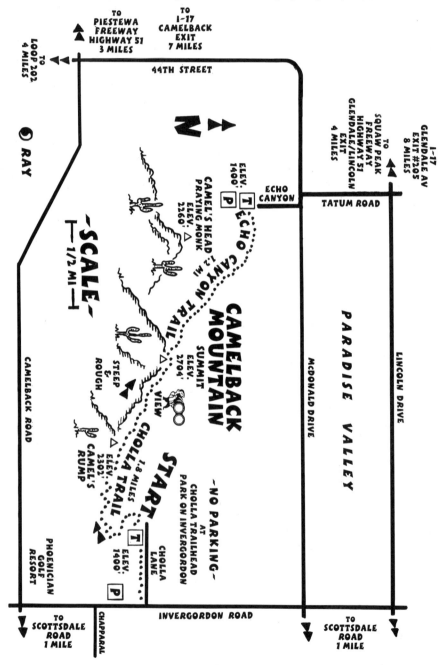

CAMELBACK MOUNTAIN
CHOLLA (SUMMIT) TRAIL

DISTANCE: 3.6 MI. TOTAL
TIME: 2-3 HOURS
EFFORT: SHORT & STEEP
TYPE: UP & DOWN
ROUTE SKILL: EASY
(SIGNED ALL THE WAY)
BEST SEASON: OCT to MAY
(HIKE VERY EXTRA EARLY IN SUMMER)
PETS: NO MUTTS ALLOWED

AT-A-GLANCE

3400

ELEV. (FT.)

1400

0   **1-WAY MILES**   1.8
(TO SUMMIT)

CHOLLA SUMMIT TRAIL
CAMELBACK

DESCRIPTION: The Camel's Back is two of the most well known hikes in Phoenix. Cholla Trail is a good choice to summit because the 1300' gain is reached over 1.8 miles, less steep than the Echo Canyon route that gains the same 1300' in only 1.2 miles. Less steep is good, right? Not always. It boils down to parking. Echo Canyon Traihead has more parking. Crowded weekends are best from Echo Canyon. Weekdays are best from the Cholla Trail end of Camelback.

The Cholla Trail hike begins from where you park down on Invergordon (See DIRECTIONS), but first you gotta walk the quarter-mile gravel path along the south side of Cholla Lane until you reach the actual trailhead kiosk. From here you quickly rise to a view of the Phoenician Resort. All that green grass and swimming look invitingly yummy.

Next the trail steeply switches up a wide ridge to the 0.8 mile mark before winding around to the cooler north side of the mountain. The less sunny, cooler, wetter north slope supports a wider variety of plant life. At mile 1.4 the trail winds back around to the east at a saddle then begins the final pitch to the summit view. A small mound to the north is Mummy Mountain. Piestewa is the big one just northwest. South Mountain and the Sierra Estrellas are to the south.

DIRECTIONS: Best approach is from I-17, Glendale Ave Exit OR from Piestewa Freeway HWY 51, Glendale Ave/Lincoln Drive Exit. Either way, head east on Glendale until it becomes Lincoln. See the map. Go right (south) on Tatum. Turn left (east) on McDonald then right (south) on Invergordon. Park the beast on the west side of Invergordon in the officially annointed areas between Cholla and Chaparral next to The Phoenician Golf Resort.

CAMELBACK
ECHO CANYON (SUMMIT) TRAIL

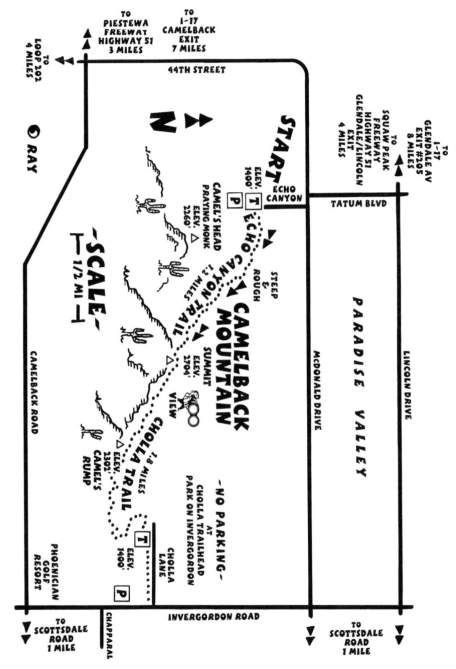

CAMELBACK MOUNTAIN
ECHO CANYON (SUMMIT) TRAIL

DISTANCE: 2.4 MI. TOTAL
TIME: 2-3 HOURS
EFFORT: SHORT & STEEP
TYPE: UP & DOWN
ROUTE SKILL: EASY
(SIGNED ALL THE WAY)
BEST SEASON: OCT to MAY
(HIKE VERY VERY EARLY IN SUMMER)
PETS: NO PETS ALLOWED

AT-A-GLANCE

2704

**ELEV.
(FT.)**

1400

0   **1-WAY MILES**   1.2
(TO SUMMIT)

FAVORITE TRAIL
WORTH A JOURNEY

ECHO CANYON SUMMIT TRAIL
CAMELBACK

DESCRIPTION: No imagination needed to spot the kneeling camel. Head and hump are clearly outlined north along the Phoenix skyline. Being the tallest of The Phoenix Mountains at 2704', the universal appeal of this sight makes it one of the most popular hikes in Arizona.

Be prepared for a short steep grunt. Summit Trail is well maintained, but you must be ready for rough terrain. Expect loose scrabble, boulders and even a few handrails to guide you up the really steep stuff. No shade. No water. No mercy.

Begin at Echo Canyon Trailhead up through Echo Canyon. Look for Praying Monk overhead. At the 0.3 mile mark you are out of the canyon and soaking the view, but the trail gets steeper and you begin to enjoy handrails up to 0.6 mile trail junction. A short detour west leads you out to a great Phoenix view along the camel's neck. Back on the main trail the hiking gets steeper and rougher up through boulder infested gullies until you peak out at 1.2 miles. Whew!

Planning a Cholla Trail "up and over" down the other side? Do-able, but have shuttle waiting at the Cholla Trailhead or face an additional 4 mile walk on city sidewalk. Ugh.

DIRECTIONS: Best approach is from Loop 101 or 202 to Piestewa Freeway HWY 51, Glendale Ave/Lincoln Drive Exit. Then head east on Lincoln. See the map. Turn RIGHT (south) on Tatum. Turn LEFT on McDonald then a quick RIGHT onto Echo Canyon Parkway to the trailhead. If too crowded, park along the east side of Echo Canyon Parkway ONLY in the few designated areas or face the con$equence$. On this hike, parking may be your biggest challenge.

LOOKOUT MOUNTAIN
SUMMIT TRAIL

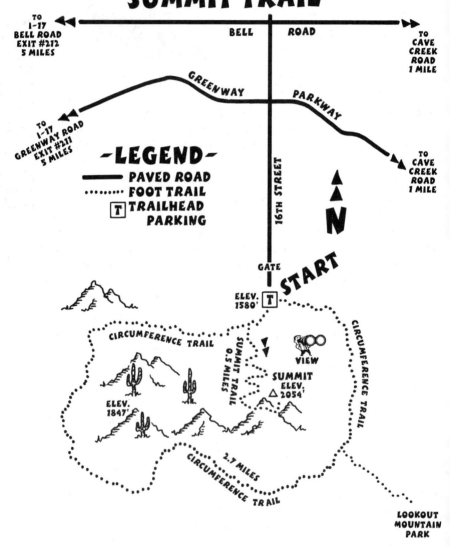

TO
I-17
BELL ROAD
EXIT #212
5 MILES

BELL   ROAD

TO
CAVE
CREEK
ROAD
1 MILE

GREENWAY   PARKWAY

TO
I-17
GREENWAY ROAD
EXIT #211
5 MILES

TO
CAVE
CREEK
ROAD
1 MILE

-LEGEND-
—— PAVED ROAD
·········· FOOT TRAIL
T TRAILHEAD
PARKING

16TH STREET

N

GATE

START

ELEV. 1580' T

CIRCUMFERENCE TRAIL

SUMMIT TRAIL 0.5 MILES

VIEW

SUMMIT ELEV. 2054'

CIRCUMFERENCE TRAIL

ELEV. 1847'

2.7 MILES
CIRCUMFERENCE TRAIL

LOOKOUT MOUNTAIN PARK

RAY

LOOKOUT MOUNTAIN
SUMMIT TRAIL TO PHOENIX PANORAMA

DISTANCE: 1 MILE TOTAL
TIME: 1 HOUR
EFFORT: SHORT & STEEP
TYPE: UP & DOWN
ROUTE SKILL: EASY
(SIGNED ALL THE WAY)
BEST SEASON: OCT to MAY
(HIKE VERY EARLY IN SUMMER)
PETS: DOGGIES ON LEASH

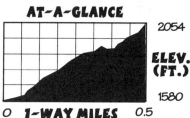

AT-A-GLANCE

2054

ELEV.
(FT.)

1580

0   1-WAY MILES   0.5
(SUMMIT TRAIL)

SUMMIT TRAIL LOOKOUT MTN

DESCRIPTION: They don't call it Lookout Mountain for nothing! Lookout is northernmost of The Phoenix Mountains that stretch like a chain of islands erupting from the sea of houses that carpets the desert floor. Shaw Butte is closest to the southwest. North Mountain is next to the south, then look for Piestewa Peak and Camelback Mountain as your eyes travel southeast. South Mountain is the one far away and due south covered with antennae. Now look far to the east and you can pick out the four distinct summits of Four Peaks. In front of them set the McDowell Mountains. This short hike to the top of Lookout Mountain is all about this unique view.

On a clear day you can pick out most city landmarks. Downtown, BOB the ballpark and Sky Harbor are due south. Tempe and ASU are southeast and you might even spot some buildings way further out in Mesa rising up out of the haze.

This hike appeals to me because it *does* get me up above the brown air layer and it does *not* have so dang many fellow hikers like other Phoenix Mountains trails. Don't count on watching the stars come out as the city lights come on though. The gate closes at sunset. No water either. The pooch must be on a leash.

Route finding is easy. There is a traihead sign near the water tower at the south end of the parking lot. After 0.1 miles Summit Trail #150 goes LEFT and Circumference Trail #308 continues right. It is a short, gradual yet relentless grade to the top. Careful not to misstep on the summit. There are sheer drops with not a soul to find your bones.

DIRECTIONS: Easy to find. From downtown, head north on I-17 going toward Flagstaff. Exit on Bell Road EAST. Continue east on Bell for 4 miles. Turn right at 16th Street and continue until the road ends in about a mile.

McDOWELL MOUNTAINS
SONORAN PRESERVE
GATEWAY TRAILS
© RAY

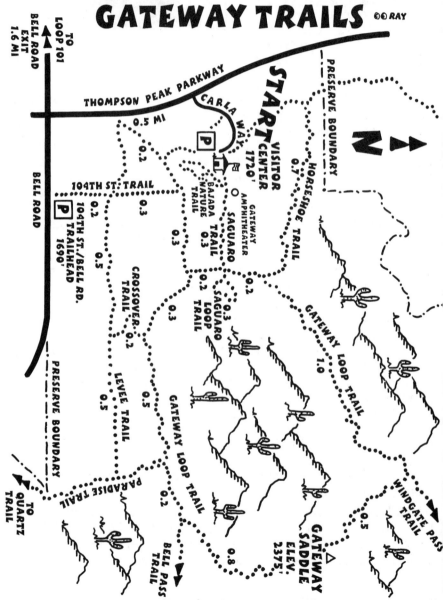

TO LOOP 101
BELL ROAD EXIT 1.6 MI

THOMPSON PEAK PARKWAY

CARLA WAY

PRESERVE BOUNDARY

START

VISITOR CENTER 1720'

BELL ROAD

0.5 MI

0.2

P

104TH ST. TRAIL

0.2

0.3

P

104TH ST./BELL RD. TRAILHEAD 1690'

0.2

0.5

HORSESHOE TRAIL

0.7

BAJADA NATURE TRAIL

GATEWAY AMPHITHEATER

SAGUARO

CROSSOVER TRAIL 0.2

0.3

0.3

0.3

SAGUARO LOOP TRAIL

0.2

0.3

0.2

0.2

GATEWAY LOOP TRAIL

1.0

LEVEE TRAIL

0.5

0.5

0.5

GATEWAY LOOP TRAIL

0.2

PRESERVE BOUNDARY

TO QUARTZ TRAIL

PARADISE TRAIL

0.8

BELL PASS TRAIL

GATEWAY SADDLE ELEV. 2375'

WINDGATE PASS TRAIL

0.5

N

McDOWELL MOUNTAINS
SONORAN DESERT PRESERVE
GATEWAY TRAILS AREA

DISTANCE: 0.5 TO 4.5 MILES
(VARIOUS TRAILS)

TIME: 1 HOUR TO ALL DAY

EFFORT: EASY TO DIFFICULT
(PLENTY OF CHOICES)

TYPE: MANY POSSIBLE LOOPS

ROUTE SKILL: EASY
(ALL TRAILS SUPER WELL SIGNED)

BEST SEASON: OCT to MAY
(HIKE ONLY EARLY AM IN SUMMER)

WILDFLOWERS: FEB to APR

PETS: ON LEASH AT ALL TIMES

The McDowell Sonoran Preserve consists of 36,400 acres set aside by the citizens of Scottsdale through the McDowell Sonoran Conservancy and supported by a voter approved sales tax. Right on Scottsdale voters! The vision is to preserve Scottsdale's natural diverse Sonoran desert habitat and create wildlife corridors to natural open spaces beyond the city for all to enjoy. FREE!

BAJADA NATURE TRAIL: 0.5 MILES/40 FEET ELEV GAIN
Very easy. Paved and wheelchair accessible interpretive tour of the diverse and amazing plants and animals living in the Sonoran desert . . . the most significant wildlife habitat in the Phoenix area. A bajada is a broad slope of debris spread across the lower slopes of mountains by descending streams. Here you can take the time to learn more about the many dozens of plant, bird and animal species who call this their home. Especially great for children.

GATEWAY LOOP: 4.5 TOTAL MILES FROM THE VISITORS CENTER/650 FEET ELEVATION GAIN
Intermediate difficulty. Allow at least two hours. No water available on the trail. Super rewarding hike up through the fabulous scenery of the McDowell Mountain foothills to Gateway Saddle where you can pause to soak up the view and catch your breath. You will have company, but not be overcrowded. If you are lucky enough to encounter wildlife, do not approach or disturb. Observe from a distance. Keep your dog on a leash for your dog's safety as well as that of the local wildlife. The preserve is open sunrise to sunset. Stay on trails. No smoking.

DIRECTIONS: Easy to find. From Loop 101 freeway in Scottsdale take the Bell Road exit. Head EAST on Bell toward the mountains for 1.6 miles. Go LEFT on Thompson Peak Pkwy for 0.5 miles and turn RIGHT into the parking area.

SONORAN PRESERVE GATEWAY
McDOWELL MTS

FAVORITE TRAIL
WORTH A JOURNEY

McDOWELL MOUNTAINS
SONORAN PRESERVE
LOST DOG TRAILS

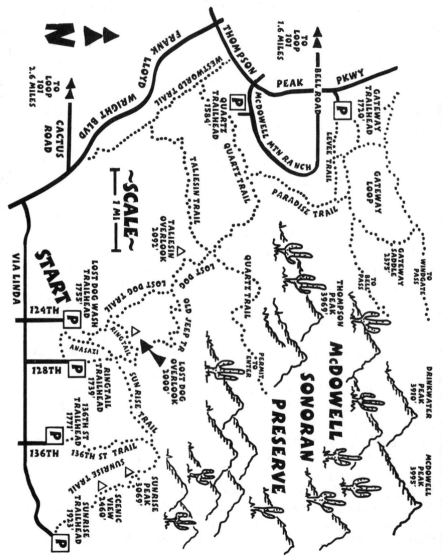

McDOWELL MOUNTAINS
SONORAN DESERT PRESERVE
LOST DOG TRAILS AREA

DISTANCE: 1.4 TO 4.9 MILES (VARIOUS TRAILS)

TIME: 1 HOUR TO ALL DAY

EFFORT: EASY TO DIFFICULT (PLENTY OF CHOICES)

TYPE: MANY LOOPS POSSIBLE

ROUTE SKILL: FAIRLY EASY (BUT NOT ALL TRAILS SIGNED)

BEST SEASON: OCT to MAY (HIKE EARLY AM IN SUMMER)

WILDFLOWERS: FEB to APR

PETS: ON LEASH AT ALL TIMES

DESCRIPTION: Everywhere you go in Scottsdale's McDowell Sonoran Preserve you can expect to be treated to a stellar experience. The Sonoran desert is alive with plants and wildlife living in harmony. Humans are the only intruder. We are guests in this alien world. Listen for birdsong. Watch for creatures scurrying or slithering in and out of view. You may encounter a rattler, a tortoise, a road runner or perhaps even a gila monster if you are very, uh, lucky. I doubt you'll encounter a lost dog in this harsh environment!

FAVORITE TRAIL ⚘ *WORTH A JOURNEY*

SONORAN PRESERVE: LOST DOG
McDOWELL MTS

The Lost Dog area at the southern end of The Preserve encompasses trails from easy to difficult. Obviously, the higher you go, the tougher it gets. The trails that roll across the bajada will be easy. Treks to a view or watch the sunrise will require some good sweaty effort. Good basic maps are available at most trailheads.

~BASIC TRAIL INFO~

LOST DOG WASH TRAIL: Easy/2.6 miles/380' elev.

OLD JEEP TRAIL: Easy/1.4 miles/192' elev. gain

RINGTAIL TRAIL: Easy/2.2 Miles/307' elev. gain

TALIESIN TRAIL: Easy/2.4 miles/431' elev. gain

QUARTZ TRAIL: Moderate/4.9 miles/1104' elev. gain

136TH STREET TRAIL: Difficult/1.6 miles/804' elev. gain

SUNRISE TRAIL: Difficult/4.4 miles/1095' elev. gain

~TRAILHEAD INFO~

LOST DOG: Good parking, water, restrooms, good signage.

RINGTAIL: Parking on west side of 128th St. No water.

SUNRISE: Parking, water, good signage, shade ramada.

QUARTZ: Park at 104th St & McDowell Ranch Rd, no water.

DIRECTIONS: From Loop 101 freeway in Scottsdale take the Cactus Road exit. Go 2.6 miles EAST toward the mountains. Turn RIGHT on Frank Lloyd Wright. Go 1 mile to Via Linda. Turn LEFT to trailheads. See map.

McDOWELL MOUNTAINS
NORTH TRAIL

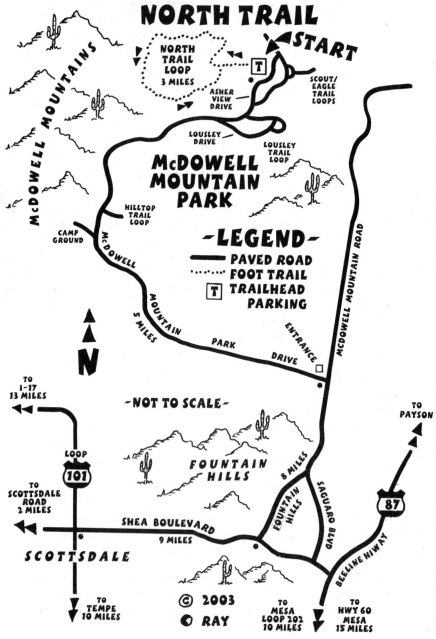

NORTH TRAIL LOOP 3 MILES

START

SCOUT/ EAGLE TRAIL LOOPS

ASHER VIEW DRIVE

LOUSLEY DRIVE

LOUSLEY TRAIL LOOP

McDOWELL MOUNTAINS

McDOWELL MOUNTAIN PARK

HILLTOP TRAIL LOOP

CAMP GROUND

McDOWELL MOUNTAIN 5 MILES

McDOWELL MOUNTAIN ROAD

~LEGEND~
— PAVED ROAD
···· FOOT TRAIL
[T] TRAILHEAD PARKING

PARK DRIVE

ENTRANCE

N

TO I-17 13 MILES

~NOT TO SCALE~

LOOP 101

TO SCOTTSDALE ROAD 2 MILES

FOUNTAIN HILLS

8 MILES

FOUNTAIN HILLS

SAGUARO BLVD

TO PAYSON

87

SHEA BOULEVARD 9 MILES

SCOTTSDALE

BEELINE HIWAY

TO TEMPE 10 MILES

© 2003 RAY

TO MESA LOOP 202 10 MILES

TO HWY 60 MESA 15 MILES

McDOWELL MOUNTAINS
NORTH TRAIL LOOP

DISTANCE: 3.1 MILES TOTAL
TIME: 2 HOURS
EFFORT: FAIRLY EASY
(NO BIG CLIMBS, BUT CROSSES WASHES)
TYPE: LOOP
ROUTE SKILL: EASY
(SIGNED, BUT STAY ON MAIN TRAIL)
BEST SEASON: OCT to MAY
(HIKE ONLY EARLY AM IN SUMMER)
WILDFLOWERS: FEB to APR

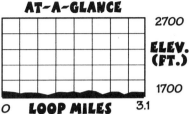

AT-A-GLANCE

2700

**ELEV.
(FT.)**

1700

O   **LOOP MILES**   3.1

PETS: DOGS ON LEASH

DESCRIPTION: In 1995, a lightning sparked wildfire roared through McDowell Mountain Park. Luckily, the area around North trail was spared along with its animal habitat. Bring binoculars. Scan holes in saguaros for owl and cactus wren nests. Watch for Harris' and red-tailed hawks, roadrunners, ravens, vultures, Gila woodpecker, cardinals and many tourist species just passing through during winter and spring. Hike early and quiet. Spot coyote, javelina, jack rabbit, antelope and lizards beyond count. Look for one BIG saguaro. I guesstimate it 50' tall. FIVE STORIES! Biggest I've seen.

Call the loop mostly flat with no big climbs, however it rolls up and down across a number of sandy washes. Once you leave the parking lot, you'll not see nor hear civilization. Except for occasional atmospheric melody of birdsong, the pervasive desert silence is almost eerie. Superb!

MILEAGE LOG

0.0   Go WEST from Palo Verde Picnic Area trailhead.
0.2   "Y" JUNCTION. Go RIGHT. Cross a several washes as you head first north, then west before looping back.
2.9   Back to "Y" JUNCTION.
3.1   Back to GO.

DIRECTIONS: From Phoenix and West Valley, take Loop Freeway 101 to Shea Blvd. See map. Exit and go EAST on Shea 9 miles to Fountain Hills. Make a LEFT on Fountain Hills Boulevard and go NORTH. CONTINUE LEFT onto McDowell Mountain Road. Make another LEFT at park entrance and CONTINUE 5 miles to LEFT at Asher View Drive South. Pull into Palo Verde Picnic Area parking. North Trail starts at the west end of the lot. From Mesa and East Valley, see the map.

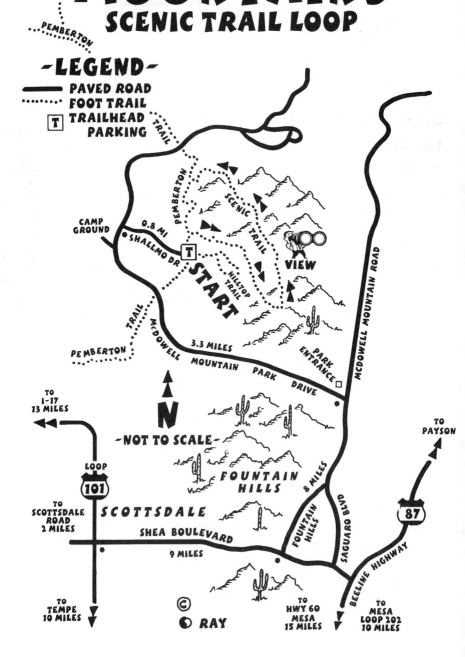

McDOWELL MOUNTAINS
SCENIC TRAIL LOOP

PEMBERTON

-LEGEND-
PAVED ROAD
FOOT TRAIL
T TRAILHEAD PARKING

PEMBERTON TRAIL

SCENIC TRAIL

CAMP GROUND

0.8 MI
SHALLMO DR

T
START

PEMBERTON TRAIL

HILLTOP TRAIL

VIEW

McDOWELL MOUNTAIN ROAD

McDOWELL MOUNTAIN PARK DRIVE

3.3 MILES

PARK ENTRANCE

PEMBERTON TRAIL

TO I-17 13 MILES

N
-NOT TO SCALE-

TO PAYSON

LOOP 101

TO SCOTTSDALE ROAD 2 MILES

SCOTTSDALE

FOUNTAIN HILLS

8 MILES

FOUNTAIN HILLS

SAGUARO BLVD

87

SHEA BOULEVARD
9 MILES

BEELINE HIGHWAY

TO TEMPE 10 MILES

© RAY

TO HWY 60 MESA 15 MILES

TO MESA LOOP 202 10 MILES

McDOWELL MOUNTAINS
SCENIC TRAIL LOOP

DISTANCE: 3.4 MILES TOTAL
TIME: 2 HOURS
EFFORT: FAIRLY EASY
TYPE: LOOP
ROUTE SKILL: EASY
(SIGNED LOOP)
BEST SEASON: OCT to MAY
(HIKE ONLY EARLY, EARLY AM IN SUMMER)
WILDFLOWERS: FEB to APR
(PEAK BLOOM MID-MARCH)

AT-A-GLANCE

2700

ELEV. (FT.)

1700

0   **LOOP MILES**   3.4

PETS: DOGS ON LEASH

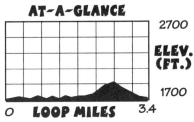

SCENIC TRAIL LOOP
McDOWELL MTS

DESCRIPTION: The 1995 lightning caused Rio Fire that roared through McDowell Mountain Park made hearts sink and cast a pall over The Valley of the Sun. Now we see the upside of fire in the desert. Wildflowers! After winter rains provide moisture, an electric bloom runs from early February to late April. Forget-me-nots, gold poppies, orange fiddleneck, globemallow, bluish-purple Coulter's lupine, brilliant yellow brittlebush and the list goes on and on. Mid-March is the absolute peak. The expansive views are great anytime.

MILEAGE LOG

0.0 From trailhead follow Pemberton Trail NORTH just a bit.
0.1 JUNCTION. Steer RIGHT onto Scenic Trail. The loop rolls up and down through washes until a short climb up a ridge to views of The Superstitions and Four Peaks east, Mazatsals north and The McDowells near west.
2.9 LEFT back onto the Pemberton Trail.
3.4 Back to the Pemberton Trailhead.

DIRECTIONS: From Phoenix and the West Valley, take Loop Freeway 101 to Shea Blvd. See the map. Exit and go EAST on Shea for 9 miles to Fountain Hills, then make a LEFT on Fountain Hills Blvd. and go NORTH 4 miles. CONTINUE LEFT onto McDowell Mountain Road 4 miles. Make another LEFT at the PARK ENTRANCE and CONTINUE 3.3 miles to SHALLMO DRIVE. RIGHT on Shallmo another 0.8 miles to the trailhead.

From Mesa and East Valley, take Superstition Freeway HWY 60 OR Loop 202 to HWY 87, Beeline Highway. Exit and go NORTH on Beeline to Shea Blvd. Go LEFT on Shea, RIGHT on Saguaro Boulevard and follow the map to the park entrance. Follow the directions above to the trailhead.

NORTH MOUNTAIN
NATIONAL (SUMMIT) TRAIL

© RAY

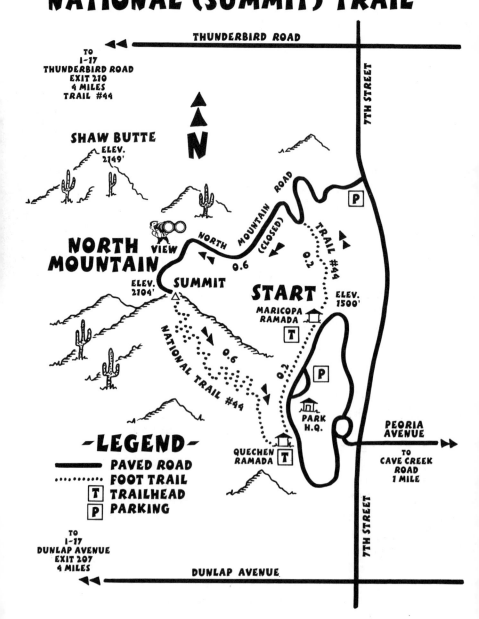

THUNDERBIRD ROAD

TO
I-17
THUNDERBIRD ROAD
EXIT 210
4 MILES
TRAIL #44

7TH STREET

N

SHAW BUTTE
ELEV.
2149'

NORTH MOUNTAIN ROAD

NORTH
MOUNTAIN
VIEW

(CLOSED)

TRAIL #44

0.6

0.2

ELEV.
2104'

SUMMIT

START

ELEV.
1500'

MARICOPA
RAMADA

T

NATIONAL TRAIL #44

0.6

0.2

P

PARK
H.Q.

PEORIA
AVENUE

TO
CAVE CREEK
ROAD
1 MILE

-LEGEND-

—————— PAVED ROAD
·········· FOOT TRAIL
T TRAILHEAD
P PARKING

QUECHEN
RAMADA

T

TO
I-17
DUNLAP AVENUE
EXIT 207
4 MILES

DUNLAP AVENUE

7TH STREET

NORTH MOUNTAIN
NATIONAL TRAIL LOOP AND VIEW

DISTANCE: 1.6 MILES TOTAL
TIME: 1 TO 1.5 HOURS
EFFORT: MODERATE
TYPE: LOOP
ROUTE SKILL: EASY
(SIGNED ALL THE WAY)
BEST SEASON: OCT to MAY
(HIKE BURLY EARLY IN SUMMER)
PETS: DOGS ON LEASH

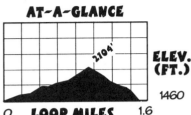

AT-A-GLANCE

2104'

ELEV. (FT.)

1460

O   **LOOP MILES**   1.6
     (NATIONAL TRAIL)

DESCRIPTION: Despite North Mountain's industrial looking, antenna infested summit and the closed-to-traffic paved service road to the top, National Trail #44 offers a fine little uncrowded loop hike as well as access to some unique views across The Valley of the Sun.

Steep and rough National Trail #44 gets rolling at the Maricopa Ramada Trailhead at the north end of the parking lot next to the ramada. From the get-go the trail goes straight up a steep draw to that closed-to-cars North Mountain Road at mile point 0.2. If you prefer pavement, you could just walk a quick up and down from the bottom of this road on 7th Street (see the map).

Anyway, proceed up the paved road. The surface is smooth, the grade is steep and there is opportunity a-plenty to breathe deep and rubber-neck the view as you walk instead of watching every step. The road comes to and end just before the summit. A Trail #44 marker indicates the last pitch to the top. Have a look around before you begin the descent. Follow rough, rocky Trail #44 down the east side of the mountain. You must now begin to seriously watch your step. The way down is quite a bit more treacherous than the ascent and easy to get rolling.

A half mile below the summit, reach a 3-way trail split. Go LEFT and drop down to Quechan Ramada. Follow Park Loop Road (see the map) a short jog back to GO.

DIRECTIONS: From I-17, take Thunderbird Road Exit #210. Head east on Thunderbird 4 miles to 7th Street. Hang a right on 7th Street. Go another 1.8 miles then turn right into the North Mountain Recreation Area Park Loop. Water and restrooms are available. The Maricopa Ramada trailhead START is at the north end of the loop.

SUMMIT LOOP TRAIL
NORTH MTN

PAPAGO PARK

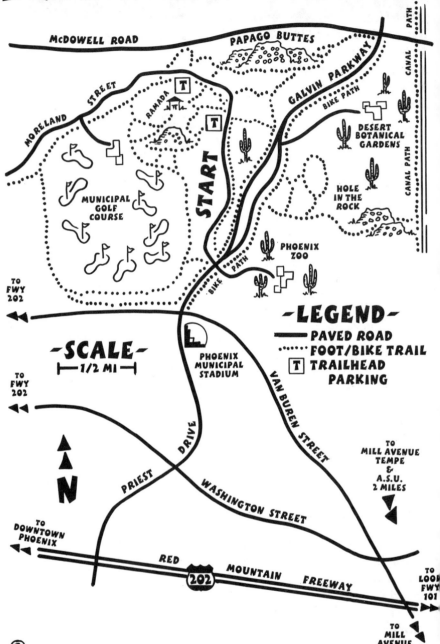

McDOWELL ROAD

PAPAGO BUTTES

MORELAND STREET

GALVIN PARKWAY

CANAL PATH

CANAL

RAMADA

BIKE PATH

START

DESERT BOTANICAL GARDENS

CANAL PATH

HOLE IN THE ROCK

MUNICIPAL GOLF COURSE

BIKE PATH

PHOENIX ZOO

TO FWY 202

-LEGEND-

SCALE

1/2 MI

— PAVED ROAD
...... FOOT/BIKE TRAIL
T TRAILHEAD PARKING

TO FWY 202

PHOENIX MUNICIPAL STADIUM

VAN BUREN STREET

N

PRIEST DRIVE

WASHINGTON STREET

TO MILL AVENUE TEMPE & A.S.U. 2 MILES

TO DOWNTOWN PHOENIX

RED MOUNTAIN FREEWAY

202

TO LOOP FWY 101

TO MILL AVENUE TEMPE

© RAY

PAPAGO PARK
LOTS OF TRAILS AND THINGS TO DO

DISTANCE: 1 - 5 MILES
TIME: 1-3 HOURS
EFFORT: NO SWEAT
TYPE: MEANDERING TRAILS
ROUTE SKILL: EASY
BEST SEASON: OCT to MAY
PETS: BRING A LEASH

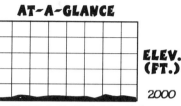

AT~A~GLANCE

ELEV. (FT.)

2000

O **5 TRAIL MILES** 5.0

DESCRIPTION: Small, dead flat, easy and smack dab in the middle of the city. Papago Park is a superb destination for folks short on time in need of a good walk over easy terrain. Not to mention that it is real close to mucho great stuff. It's easy to burn an hour or a whole day here.

A more or less informal trail system runs helter skelter over the whole 1200 acres. Some are signed. Most are not. If you orient yourself to the big buttes, you can't get lost. I like to loop around the larger buttes, maybe cut over to Hole in the Rock and then head into the zoo if I have my kids along. Otherwise, I might check out the Desert Botanical Garden or catch a baseball game at Muni Stadium if the Oakland As are in town for spring training. After that, I might hoof it over to Mill Avenue for a tall latte and a treat at The Plantation or maybe a sandwich accompanied by a frosty adult beverage at one of the many local watering holes. See what I mean. Lots to do. Bring water. Bring money.

The park, open sunrise to sunset, includes ramadas, grills, bathrooms, fishing lagoons, a pyramid (actually a tomb), a golf course and lots and lots of bike paths. And did I say bike paths? Beware the plague, the pox, the ides and the rookies out on mountain bike rides. Easy trails run amok, all too perfect for the novice mountain biker. Most are friendly and polite. A few are fast, rude and reckless. Stay out of their way and let Darwin do his work.

By the way, in case you're wondering about in the rocks, the red rock buttes (iron oxide-hematite) were formed 6 to 15 million years ago. The swiss cheese holes, called tafoni, were formed by water breaking up minerals in the rock.

DIRECTIONS: From Loop 202, Red Mountain Freeway, take the Van Buren exit. Go east about one mile to the Galvin Parkway, turn left into Papago Park then see the map.

"The time you enjoy wasting is not wasted time."
T.S. Eliot

PHOENIX MOUNTAINS
CHRISTIANSEN TRAIL #100

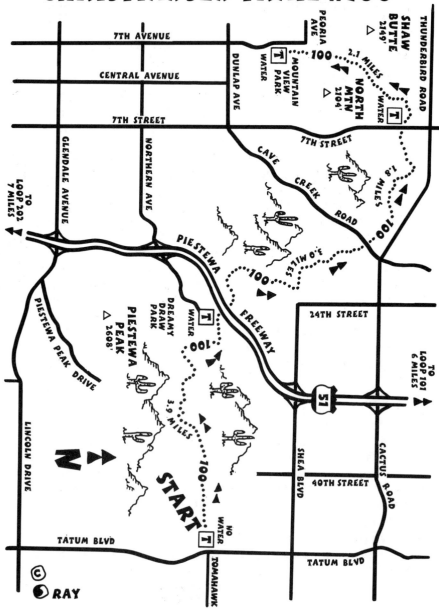

7TH AVENUE

CENTRAL AVENUE

7TH STREET

DUNLAP AVE

PEORIA AVE

WATER

MOUNTAIN VIEW PARK

100

2.1 MILES

SHAW BUTTE 2149'

THUNDERBIRD ROAD

NORTH MTN 2104'

WATER

7TH STREET

GLENDALE AVENUE

NORTHERN AVE

TO LOOP 202 7 MILES

CAVE CREEK ROAD

1.8 MILES 100

PIESTEWA

3.0 MILES

100

DREAMY DRAW PARK

PIESTEWA PEAK 2608'

WATER

100

FREEWAY

24TH STREET

TO LOOP 101 6 MILES

51

PIESTEWA PEAK DRIVE

3.9 MILES

100

START

SHEA BLVD

40TH STREET

CACTUS ROAD

LINCOLN DRIVE

N

NO WATER

TATUM BLVD

TOMAHAWK

TATUM BLVD

© RAY

PHOENIX MOUNTAINS
CHRISTIANSEN TRAIL #100

DISTANCE: 10.8 MILES
TIME: ALL DAY
EFFORT: ITSA LONG WAY
TYPE: SHUTTLE
ROUTE SKILL: EASY
(SIGNED ALL THE WAY)
BEST SEASON: OCT to MAY
(WAY TOO HOT IN SUMMER)
WILDFLOWERS: FEB to APR
(PEAK SEASON MARCH)

AT-A-GLANCE

2300

ELEV. (FT.)

1300

0   **1-WAY MILES**   10.8

PETS: MUTTS ON LEASH
(PHOENIX PARKS LAW)

DESCRIPTION: I am always amazed how I can be hiking a trail in the proverbial belly of the beast, beast in this case being City of Phoenix, yet feel as though I am at home in the middle of nowhere. Miles of silent trail through perfect Sonoran Desert is interrupted only every so often by a tunnel passing under a major urban arterial. Then just as suddenly, the city vanishes, the roar of traffic fades and I am back in my reverie. Very cool! The Phoenix Mountains cut a swath across the heart of the city. Trail #100 connects the dots through this mountain range from end to end, coast to coast.

Clearly marked all the way. After leaving the ultra-tiny undeveloped trailhead on Tatum (see the map) you can count on finding water and bathrooms at each of the subsequent trailheads along the way. Despite rolling through some wicked tough topography, Trail #100 prefers to roll *around* mountains rather than *over* them. Long story short, this superb trail has its ups and downs, but nothing too serious, steep or rough. The western end might be considered a tad bleak, but the entire rest is most excellent with the area east of Dreamy Draw best for scenery, flowers and cacti. Lots of speedy mountain bikers on weekends.

Due to the length, a shuttle full of frosty pops waiting at the end will be most welcome. East to west is best. The trailhead on Tatum is dinky. Don't count on parking a vehicle there.

DIRECTIONS: From Loop 101 or 202, get on HWY 51 to the Shea Blvd. Exit. Go 2 miles EAST on Shea to Tatum Blvd. RIGHT on Tatum for just over a mile and the tiny trailhead is on your RIGHT just across from an equally tiny street named Tomahawk Trail. Don't blink or you might miss it.

PICACHO PEAK
SUMMIT TRAILS

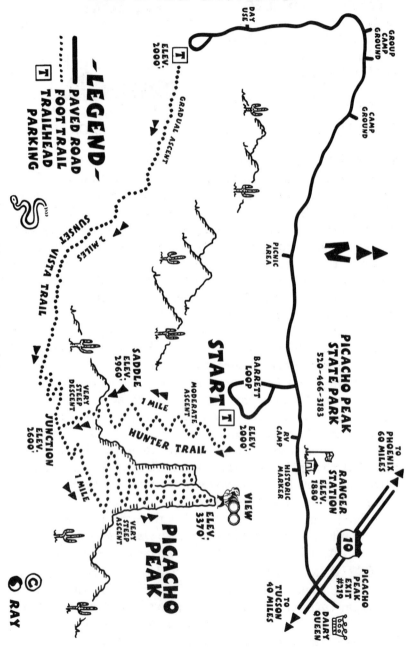

-LEGEND-
- ━━━ PAVED ROAD
- ········ FOOT TRAIL
- T TRAILHEAD PARKING

DAY USE

ELEV. 2000'

GROUP CAMP GROUND

CAMP GROUND

GRADUAL ASCENT

2 MILES

SUNSET VISTA TRAIL

PICNIC AREA

N

PICACHO PEAK STATE PARK
520-466-3183

BARRETT LOOP

START

T ELEV. 2000'

SADDLE ELEV. 2960'

MODERATE ASCENT

1 MILE

HUNTER TRAIL

VERY STEEP DESCENT

JUNCTION ELEV. 2600'

1 MILE

VIEW
ELEV. 3370'

VERY STEEP ASCENT

PICACHO PEAK

RV CAMP

HISTORIC MARKER

RANGER STATION ELEV. 1880'

TO PHOENIX 60 MILES

10

PICACHO PEAK EXIT #219

DAIRY QUEEN

TO TUCSON 40 MILES

© RAY

DISTANCE: 4 MILES TOTAL
TIME: 3-4 HOURS
EFFORT: NO MERCY
TYPE: UP & DOWN
ROUTE SKILL: EASY
(SIGNED ALL THE WAY)
BEST SEASON: OCT to MAY
WILDFLOWERS: FEB to APR
(PEAK SEASON MARCH)

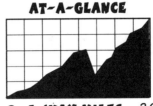

AT-A-GLANCE

3370

ELEV. (FT.)

2000

O   **1-WAY MILES**   2.0
(VIA HUNTER TRAIL)

DESCRIPTION: Picacho is so steep you will question your sanity while holding on for dear life to cables bolted into sheer rock. This is a no dog hike. Fifi would hate you. The summit is an epic adrenaline pumping adventure to remember.

FAVORITE TRAIL

WORTH A JOURNEY

My *Roadside Geology* tells me that "ship-of-the-desert" Picacho Peak is not a volcanic neck as it appears, but "the faulted, tilted and eroded remains of a series of lava flows. The summit contains a single block of granite that was ripped from the wall of a lava conduit and carried to the surface". Wow!

Hike early. Hunter Trail climbs the morning shaded side of Picacho. Start uphill right away to "The Saddle" where you grab a cable and head steep down for a couple of hundred feet. Quickly meet the junction of Sunset Vista Trail and then things get seriously steep up all the way to the summit. This whole business up to the top is only 2 miles one way, but may take 2 hours up and an hour down not counting time outs for heavy breathing.

A somewhat easier, longer alternative is to approach the junction of Hunter and Sunset Vista via Sunset Vista Trail. See the map. At 3.1 miles one way, it is more gradual at first without a trip up over "The Saddle", but you still do the very serious last bit to the top.

Bring sturdy shoes, lots of water, good snacks, a hat, light gloves for the many steel cable sections and leave the walking stick home. You're gonna need both hands.

DIRECTIONS: Easy. It's right on I-10 between Phoenix and Tucson. See the map. What is most amazing to me is how they put it right next to a Dairy Queen. You will no doubt require a large Rambo Blizzard after your Picacho summit.

SUMMIT TRAILS
PICACHO PEAK

PINNACLE PEAK

PINNACLE PEAK TRAIL

(CITY OF SCOTTSDALE)

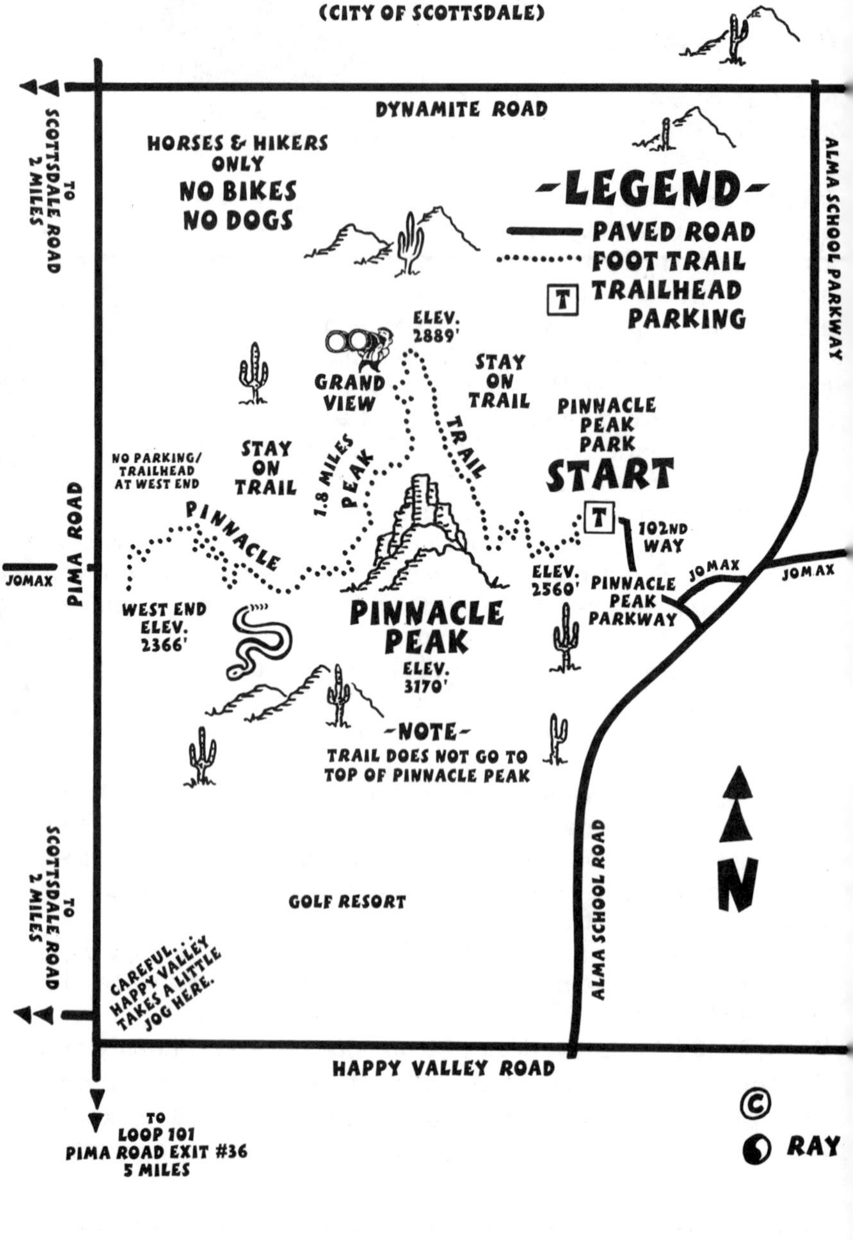

DYNAMITE ROAD

TO SCOTTSDALE ROAD 2 MILES

ALMA SCHOOL PARKWAY

HORSES & HIKERS ONLY
NO BIKES
NO DOGS

-LEGEND-
PAVED ROAD
FOOT TRAIL
T TRAILHEAD PARKING

ELEV. 2889'

GRAND VIEW

STAY ON TRAIL

PINNACLE PEAK PARK
START

NO PARKING/ TRAILHEAD AT WEST END

STAY ON TRAIL

1.8 MILES

PINNACLE PEAK

TRAIL

PINNACLE

PIMA ROAD

JOMAX

T 102ND WAY

JOMAX

JOMAX

ELEV. 2560'

PINNACLE PEAK PARKWAY

WEST END ELEV. 2366'

PINNACLE PEAK
ELEV. 3170'

-NOTE-
TRAIL DOES NOT GO TO TOP OF PINNACLE PEAK

ALMA SCHOOL ROAD

N

TO SCOTTSDALE ROAD 2 MILES

GOLF RESORT

CAREFUL. HAPPY VALLEY TAKES A LITTLE JOG HERE.

HAPPY VALLEY ROAD

TO LOOP 101 PIMA ROAD EXIT #36 5 MILES

© RAY

PINNACLE PEAK
PINNACLE PEAK TRAIL

DISTANCE: 1.75 MILES 1-WAY
TIME: 1.5 to 2 HOURS
EFFORT: EASY to MEDIUM
FAIRLY SMOOTH BUT ROLLING TERRAIN
TYPE: OUT & BACK
ROUTE SKILL: EASY
LOTS OF SIGNS
BEST SEASON: OCT to MAY
HIKE DAWN OR DUSK IN SUMMER
WILDFLOWERS: JAN to APR **PETS:** NO DOGS

AT-A-GLANCE

3300

ELEV. (FT.)

2300

O **1-WAY MILES** 1.75

DESCRIPTION: Pinnacle Peak is quite the sight. You can't help but stare for a spell. The granite spire has long been a magnet for hikers and climbers. Luxury homes and resorts surrounded the peak in the 1990s, but Pinnacle Peak Park once again opened to the public in 2002.

Pinnacle Peak Trail offers a superb desert experience without being really remote. Horses and hikers share the trail as well as climbers headed up the peak. Poppies and lupines go off around the first of the year and continue all spring. Cactus flowers go full bright electric in April.

Please stay on the trail. Private property surrounds the park. Owners are finicky about you being in their back yard. Same goes for the desert wildlife and vegetation. Stay on trail and everybody will be happy.

Crowded on weekends. Bathrooms, water and parking for 50 cars at the trailhead. Good interpretive signs along the way, but no water. Wear sturdy shoes and protection from the sun. Carry some water. Watch out for rattlers.

DIRECTIONS: Pinnacle Peak is located in far north Scottsdale on the northwest flank of the McDowell Mountains. From downtown Scottsdale, go NORTH on Scottsdale Road to Happy Valley Road. Turn RIGHT and head EAST on Happy Valley 3 miles to Alma School Road. Go LEFT on Alma School another mile until you see signs to Pinnacle Peak and Pinnacle Peak Patio Restaurant on the LEFT.

From anywhere else in The Valley, it's easy to get here and easy to find thanks to Loop Freeway 101. Just take 101 to Pima Road Exit #36. Then head NORTH on Pima Road for 5 miles. Take a RIGHT on Happy Valley. LEFT on Alma School and LEFT on Pinnacle Peak Parkway. See the map.

PINNACLE PEAK TRAIL
PINNACLE PEAK

SHAW BUTTE LOOP
SUMMIT LOOP TRAIL

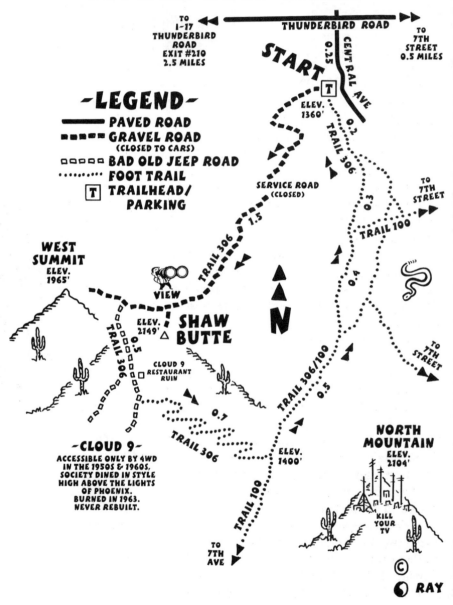

TO
I-17
THUNDERBIRD
ROAD
EXIT #210
2.5 MILES

THUNDERBIRD ROAD

TO
7TH
STREET
0.5 MILES

START

CENTRAL AVE

0.25

T

ELEV.
1360'

0.2

TRAIL 306

0.3

TO
7TH
STREET

TRAIL 100

-LEGEND-
— PAVED ROAD
▪▪▪▪▪ GRAVEL ROAD
(CLOSED TO CARS)
▢▢▢▢▢ BAD OLD JEEP ROAD
.... FOOT TRAIL
T TRAILHEAD/
PARKING

SERVICE ROAD
(CLOSED)

1.5

TRAIL 306

0.4

WEST
SUMMIT
ELEV.
1965'

VIEW

ELEV.
2149' △

SHAW
BUTTE

▲▲
▲
N

TRAIL 306

0.5

CLOUD 9
RESTAURANT
RUIN

TRAIL 306/100

0.5

TO
7TH
STREET

0.7

NORTH
MOUNTAIN
ELEV.
2104'

-CLOUD 9-
ACCESSIBLE ONLY BY 4WD
IN THE 1950S & 1960S.
SOCIETY DINED IN STYLE
HIGH ABOVE THE LIGHTS
OF PHOENIX.
BURNED IN 1963.
NEVER REBUILT.

TRAIL 306

ELEV.
1400'

TRAIL 100

KILL
YOUR
TV

TO
7TH
AVE

© RAY

SHAW BUTTE LOOP
LOOP TRAIL #306 TO SUMMIT VIEWS

DISTANCE: 4.1 MILES TOTAL
TIME: 2 TO 3 HOURS
EFFORT: MODERATE
TYPE: LOOP TO SUMMIT
ROUTE SKILL: EASY
(SIGNED ALL THE WAY)
BEST SEASON: OCT to MAY
(HIKE ZERO-DARK-30 IN SUMMER)
WILDFLOWERS: FEB to APR
(PEAK SEASON MARCH)

AT-A-GLANCE

2149'

ELEV.
(FT.)
1360

0   **LOOP MILES**   4.1
(VIA TRAIL #306)

PETS: DOGS ON LEASH

DESCRIPTION: Great loop hike in the northernmost part of Phoenix Mountains Preserve. BEST DONE COUNTER-CLOCK-WISE to hike *up* a fairly smooth service road to the towers and summit and then descend the gnarly stuff. Hard to get lost with all the Trail #306 markers. Shaw Butte is under your feet at first for the up-and-over and then over your left shoulder as you circle back to the trailhead. On top, don't miss the short side hike to the towers and bragging rights to the actual summit.

Yellow brittlebush flowers set the mountain on fire with color after a rainy winter. A slightly shadier and cooler north side of Shaw Butte supports an abundant variety of Sonoran Desert vegetation. You'll want sturdy shoes for the rough stuff, plenty of water and possibly a good snack.

MILEAGE LOG

0.0 Parking and Trailhead. Head up service road.
1.4 Left to summit or CONTINUE RIGHT on TR #306.
1.5 Saddle. Go LEFT thru steel pipe barriers. Continue as you keep a sharp eye for TR #306 markers.
2.0 Sharp LEFT onto trail marked TR #306 heading down just after burned out *Cloud 9 Restaurant* ruin.
2.7 LEFT onto TR #306/#100. A sharp eye here for signs. Many trails try to confuse. See the map.
3.2 CONTINUE on #306 back to trailhead.
4.1 Back to GO.

DIRECTIONS: Quickest way to get here from almost any-where in Phoenix is to take I-17 to Thunderbird Road Exit #210. Head east on Thunderbird for 2.5 miles to Central. Take a right on Central and go south for only a quarter mile. Parking area and trailhead on the right.

SHAW BUTTE

SOUTH MOUNTAIN
ALTA/BAJADA LOOP TRAIL

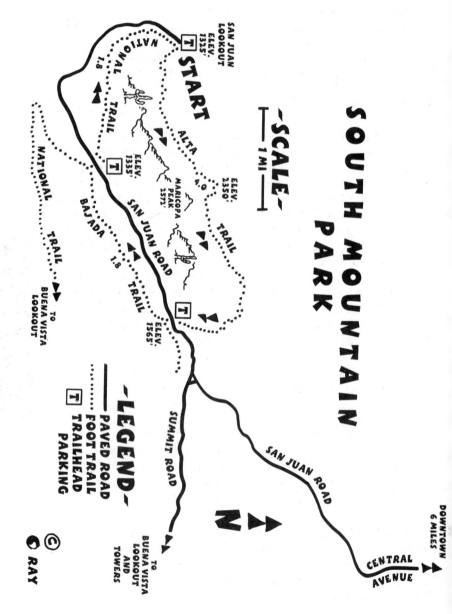

SOUTH MOUNTAIN PARK

START

SAN JUAN LOOKOUT ELEV. 1325'

NATIONAL TRAIL 1.8

ELEV. 1335'

MARICOPA PEAK 2571'

ALTA TRAIL 4.0

ELEV. 2350'

NATIONAL TRAIL TO BUENA VISTA LOOKOUT

BAJADA TRAIL 1.8

SAN JUAN ROAD

ELEV. 1565'

-SCALE-
1 MI

SUMMIT ROAD

TO BUENA VISTA LOOKOUT AND TOWERS

SAN JUAN ROAD

CENTRAL AVENUE

DOWNTOWN 6 MILES

N

-LEGEND-
—— PAVED ROAD
..... FOOT TRAIL
T TRAILHEAD PARKING

© RAY

SOUTH MOUNTAIN
ALTA/BAJADA LOOP

DISTANCE: 7.6 MILES TOTAL
TIME: ALLOW 4 to 5 HOURS
EFFORT: HARSH
TYPE: LONG LOOP
ROUTE SKILL: EASY
(SIGNED ALL THE WAY)
BEST SEASON: OCT to MAY
(TOO DAMN HOT IN SUMMER)
WILDFLOWERS: FEB to APR
(PEAK SEASON MARCH)

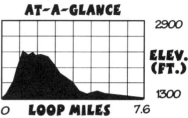

AT-A-GLANCE

2900

ELEV.
(FT.)

1300

0   LOOP MILES   7.6

PETS: DOG ON LEASH

DESCRIPTION: Sheesh. This hike really kicked my butt one fine warm January day. Sort of like eating a cheap steak. Tough as toenails, but once you finish at least you know you ate something. Nobody goes out here. Real quiet high above the city. You'll be all alone. You might like it. I did.

Goes straight up 1,000 feet ascending a ridgeline in the very first very long mile, then down and up just a bit and finally home free descending most of the return. The Alta/Bajada Loop is a longish 7.6 miles and arguably the toughest loop at South Mountain. There is no water. Carry at least a gallon any time of year. jjggThe trail is rough and rocky, but you are hiking trailhead to trailhead with little chance of becoming lost.

MILEAGE LOG

0.0 You might hate me for this. ALTA TRAIL is UP and steep at first, but mellows out in about a mile and a quarter. Then go down and up just a bit for another mile and a half before things really get rolling downhill.

4.0 SAN jUAN ROAD and JUNCTION with Bajada Trail. Cross the road and Go RIGHT on Bajada.

5.8 JUNCTION with National Trail. Go RIGHT on National across San Juan Road and CONTINUE following National as it parallels San Juan Road all the way home.

7.6 Back to GO safe, sound and well tuckered.

DIRECTIONS: From downtown Phoenix go 6 miles SOUTH on Central Avenue STRAIGHT into South Mountain Park. Continue all the way up to the JUNCTION with Summit Road and San Juan Road. Go RIGHT on SAN JUAN ROAD and all the way to SAN JUAN LOOKOUT at the very end of the road. Leave no valuables in your car to tempt the bad guys.

ALTA/BAJADA LOOP TRAIL
SOUTH MTN

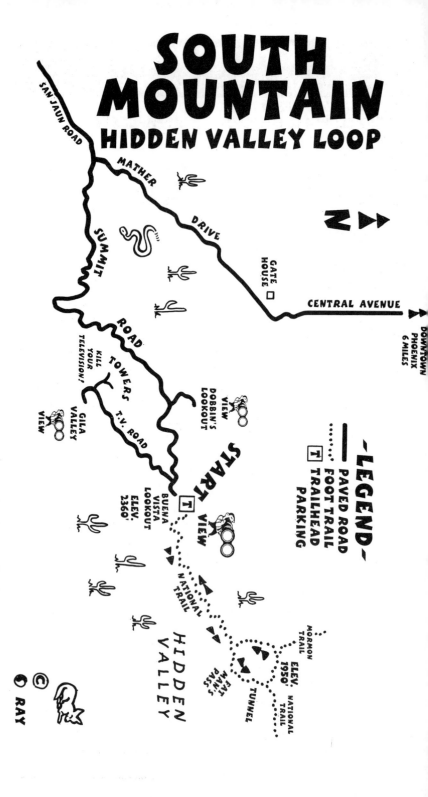

SOUTH MOUNTAIN
VIEWS FROM A *HIDDEN VALLEY*

DISTANCE: 3.5 MILES TOTAL
TIME: 2 to 3 HOURS
EFFORT: MODERATE
TYPE: OUT & BACK, SORTA
ROUTE SKILL: EASY
(SIGNED MOST OF THE WAY)
BEST SEASON: OCT to MAY
WILDFLOWERS: FEB to APR

AT~A~GLANCE

2900

ELEV. (FT.)

1900

O   **TOTAL MILES**   3.5

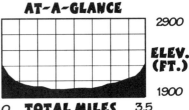

DESCRIPTION: Short, moderate hike. Not steep. Good trail. Well marked. Close to town. Brilliant flowers in season. Superb cactus collection. Views in every direction. What could be better? Avoid weekends! During good weather, you can't swing a dead cat without hitting a hiker or mountain biker. Most cyclists are polite and will go out of their way to share the trail, but there is always the exception. As a hiker, you have right-of-way, but be warned. Weekdays best. Watch your step. Wear a hat. Carry water.

MILEAGE LOG

0.0   Kick off your hike from the Buena Vista Lookout down National Trail. You follow along a ridge at first, soaking up views of the city and distant desert mountain ranges. Careful not to brush against the evil cholla as you enjoy the hedgehog and saguaro. If you're lucky and there has been some rain, the sticks of the ocotillo will be leafy green topped with a red bloom. Brittlebush will line your path with brilliant yellow flowers. Beautiful.

1.5   Turn RIGHT at Hidden Valley sign. If you can't clear Fatman's Pass (not *that* narrow), see a doctor. Next check out more passages in the boulders, The Window and The Natural Tunnel.

1.7   Just after The Tunnel, Hidden Valley spur rejoins National. Go LEFT, then stay LEFT at Mormon Trail and head back up National Trail to Buena Vista Lookout.

3.5   Whew. Hope you left something cool cooling in the cooler.

DIRECTIONS: From downtown Phoenix, go due south on Central Avenue for 6 miles. Central leads directly into South Mountain Park. As soon as you enter the park you start heading UP. From there, easy as heck to follow the map.

SOUTH MOUNTAIN
HOLBERT TRAIL
TO
DOBBINS LOOKOUT

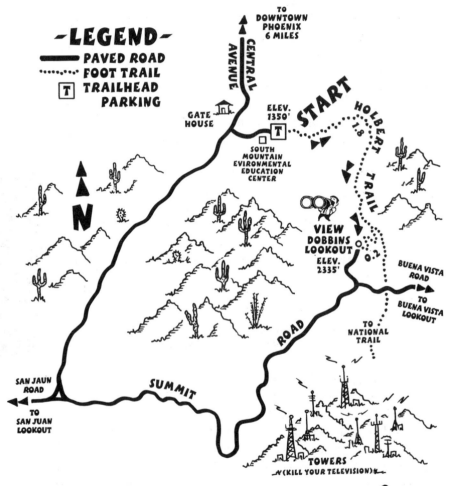

-LEGEND-

⎯⎯⎯ PAVED ROAD
············ FOOT TRAIL
[T] TRAILHEAD PARKING

TO DOWNTOWN PHOENIX 6 MILES

CENTRAL AVENUE

GATE HOUSE

ELEV. 1350' [T]

START

HOLBERT 1.8 TRAIL

SOUTH MOUNTAIN EVIRONMENTAL EDUCATION CENTER

N

VIEW DOBBINS LOOKOUT ELEV. 2335'

0.2

BUENA VISTA ROAD

TO BUENA VISTA LOOKOUT

TO NATIONAL TRAIL

SUMMIT ROAD

SAN JAUN ROAD

TO SAN JUAN LOOKOUT

TOWERS
(KILL YOUR TELEVISION)

©

 RAY

SOUTH MOUNTAIN
HOLBERT TRAIL TO DOBBINS LOOKOUT

DISTANCE: 4.0 MILES TOTAL
TIME: 3 HOURS
EFFORT: TOUGH
(STEEP CLIMB, STEEP DESCENT)
TYPE: OUT & BACK
ROUTE SKILL: EASY
(SIGNED ALL THE WAY)
BEST SEASON: OCT to MAY
WILDFLOWERS: FEB to APR

AT-A-GLANCE

2350

ELEV. (FT.)

1350

O **TOTAL MILES** 4.0

PETS: DOGS ON LEASH

DESCRIPTION: Dobbins Lookout, at the top of Summit Road, is the most impressive New Deal lookout structure at South Mountain. Built by the Civilian Conservation Corps in 1938, the lookout was named for Jim Dobbins, who in 1924 had the foresight to convince the City of Phoenix to purchase South Mountain, preserve the area as a park and thus save it from destructive mining operations. The CCC built several trails and lookouts at South Mountain during the depths of The Great Depression. Hand built out of local granite rubble, these shelters look like natural rock outcroppings and imitate the appearance of South Mountain's natural peaks. The rough edged stone adds to this effect. Beautiful!

MILEAGE LOG

0.0 From Holbert Trailhead the route is flat for the first half mile or so, then heads up steep and gets steeper.

1.8 Go steep RIGHT up to Dobbins Lookout.

2.0 Dobbins Lookout. Congratulations. Hope you brought the binocs. Catch your breath, have a snack, look around and head back down the way you came.

4.0 Back to GO. Stop in at SMEEC. They are full of great South Mountain info regarding trails, hiking, biking, F.D.R.'s 1930s New Deal architecture and more.

DIRECTIONS: From downtown Phoenix, go due SOUTH on Central Avenue for 6 miles. Central leads directly into South Mountain Park. As you enter the park, take the first LEFT after the GATEHOUSE. Park at the South Mountain Environmental Education Center and then walk a short bit east to the trailhead. Your car is safe here, but lock goodies out of sight so as not to tempt any roaming goofballs.

HOLBERT TRAIL
SOUTH MTN

SOUTH MOUNTAIN
JAVELINA/BEVERLY CANYON LOOP

© RAY

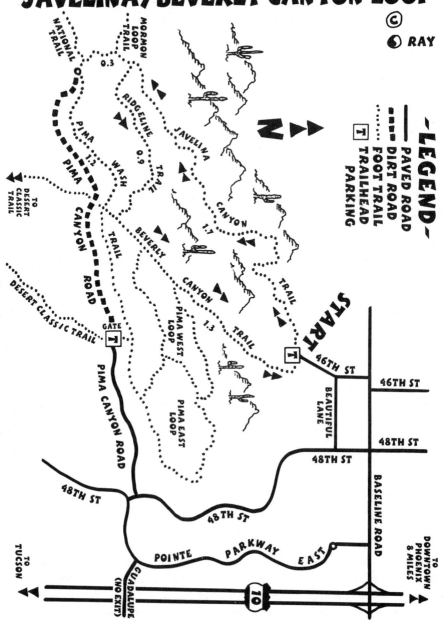

-LEGEND-

— PAVED ROAD
- - - DIRT ROAD
.... FOOT TRAIL
T TRAILHEAD PARKING

N ▶▶

NATIONAL TRAIL

MORMON LOOP TRAIL

0.3

RIDGELINE 0.9

PIMA 1.2

PIMA WASH

JAVELINA TRAIL

PIMA CANYON ROAD

TO DESERT CLASSIC TRAIL

DESERT CLASSIC TRAIL

BEVERLY CANYON LOOP

1.7

CANYON

1.3

TRAIL

GATE T

PIMA WEST LOOP

PIMA EAST LOOP

PIMA CANYON ROAD

START T

46TH ST

46TH ST

BEAUTIFUL LANE

48TH ST

48TH ST

48TH ST

48TH ST

POINTE PARKWAY EAST

BASELINE ROAD

TO DOWNTOWN PHOENIX 8 MILES

TO TUCSON

GUADALUPE (NO EXIT)

10

SOUTH MOUNTAIN
JAVELINA/BEVERLY CANYON LOOP

DISTANCE: 3.9 MILES TOTAL
TIME: 2 HOURS
EFFORT: EASY TO MEDIUM
TYPE: UP AND DOWN LOOP
ROUTE SKILL: FAIRLY EASY
(SIGNED ALL THE WAY)
BEST SEASON: OCT to MAY
(HIKE ONLY VERY EARLY AM IN SUMMER)
PETS: POOCH ON LEASH

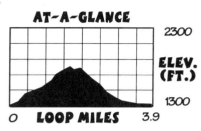

AT-A-GLANCE

2300

ELEV. (FT.)

1300

0   LOOP MILES   3.9

DESCRIPTION: Javelina are a type of wild pig common to the desert southwest. They get to be the size of a large dog. They do not have tusks nor can they see all that well, but they do have rather large yellow teeth and smell pretty bad. They travel in small herds and can be aggressive when cornered or threatened. Speaking from my own personal experience, I have never seen one on Javelina Canyon Trail, however you do not want to be the object of their attention. They are quite tasty stewed with southwestern spices and fresh veggies. I have no experience with anyone named Beverly.

Javelina Canyon/Beverly Canyon Loop is moderately easy and fairly well signed. The surrounding Sonoran Desert in the eastern foothills of South Mountain is pretty and uncrowded. The views from Ridgeline Trail are excellent.

MILEAGE LOG

0.0 After making sure that you have a good supply of water, head up Javelina Canyon Trail. Not very steep here.

1.7 Go LEFT onto Ridgeline Trail and begin short steep climb up to a ridge. Once on top, the trail rolls over four small summits. You've only climbed about 400', but fine views expand across the flat expanse of Phoenix, Sky Harbor, downtown and several desert sky islands.

2.6 LEFT onto Beverly Canyon Trail and follow all the way back to the trailhead.

3.9 Back to Beverly Canyon Trailhead.

DIRECTIONS: From downtown Phoenix go SOUTH on I-10 in direction of Tucson for about 8 miles. Take Baseline Road exit and go WEST about a mile to 46th Street. Go LEFT on 46th and CONTINUE toward South Mountain to Beverly Canyon Trailhead at end of the road. Leave no valuables in your car.

"Not one shred of evidence supports the notion that life is serious."
-Anon

JAVELINA LOOP
SOUTH MTN

SOUTH MOUNTAIN
KIWANIS/RANGER TRAIL LOOP

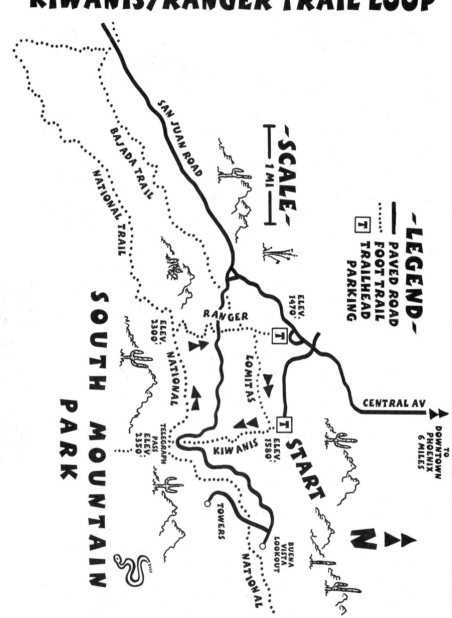

SOUTH MOUNTAIN
KIWANIS/RANGER LOOP TRAIL

DISTANCE: 4.2 MILES TOTAL
TIME: 2 TO 3 HOURS
EFFORT: MEDIUM
TYPE: UP & DOWN LOOP
ROUTE SKILL: FAIRLY EASY
(SIGNED ALL THE WAY)
BEST SEASON: OCT to MAY
(HIKE ONLY VERY EARLY AM IN SUMMER)
WILDFLOWERS: FEB to APR
(PEAK SEASON MARCH)

AT-A-GLANCE

2500

**ELEV.
(FT.)**

1500

0   **LOOP MILES**   4.2

PETS: POOCH ON LEASH

DESCRIPTION: At night, the blinking red lights of South Mountain's towers define the southern horizon of Phoenix. South Mountain Park & Preserve covers 16,500 acres and is the largest city park in America. 3 million people come every year to hike and bike. Ranger/Kiwanis Loop is a rugged, quick and uncrowded ascent to the mountain's east-west ridgeline and return. Shortly after a wet winter, colorful flowers on this north facing slope cannot be beat. Start with a very steep 700' climb in the first mile to the ridgeline and the rest of the loop is a breeze. The views along the ridge are stellar.

MILEAGE LOG

0.0   Head straight UP old Indian trade route Kiwanis Trail through Snake Canyon to National Trail at ridgeline. Mellow at first, but gets steep quick. If your timing is right, you'll enjoy lots of brilliant gold poppies, yellowish-orange fiddleneck and bright yellow brittlebush flowers.

1.0   Cross Summit Road to National Trail JUNCTION at Telegraph Pass. Go RIGHT and west along the ridgeline walking the spine of South Mountain. Views aplenty.

2.3   JUNCTION with Ranger Trail. Go RIGHT and down. Again, steep at first then levels out.

3.3   JUNCTION with Bajada Trail. Continue down Ranger.

3.5   RIGHT on Los Lomitas Trail back to Kiwanis Trailhead.

4.2   Finish. For a shorter hike just hike up and down either Kiwanis or Ranger.

DIRECTIONS: From downtown Phoenix, go due south on Central Avenue for 6 miles. Central leads directly into South Mountain Park. Continue another 0.6 miles past the park entrance to a LEFT at a signed turnoff. Go another 0.7 miles to the Kiwanis Trailhead. Park and head up Kiwanis Trail.

**KIWANIS/RANGER LOOP
SOUTH MTN**

SOUTH MOUNTAIN
NATIONAL/MORMON LOOP

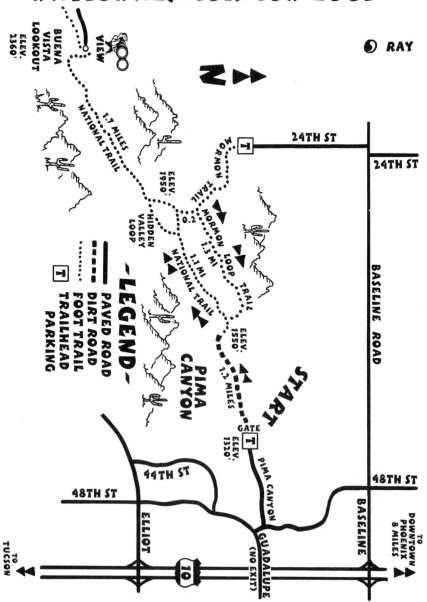

RAY

BUENA VISTA LOOKOUT
ELEV. 2360'

VIEW

1.7 MILES
NATIONAL TRAIL

24TH ST

24TH ST

MORMON TRAIL

ELEV. 1950'

0.2

HIDDEN VALLEY LOOP

MORMON LOOP TRAIL

1.3 MI

1.1 MI
NATIONAL TRAIL

ELEV. 1550'

BASELINE ROAD

-LEGEND-

PAVED ROAD
DIRT ROAD
FOOT TRAIL
TRAILHEAD
PARKING

PIMA CANYON

1.2 MILES

START

GATE
ELEV. 1320'

44TH ST

48TH ST

48TH ST

ELLIOT

PIMA CANYON

BASELINE

TO DOWNTOWN PHOENIX 8 MILES

TO TUCSON

10

GUADALUPE (NO EXIT)

SOUTH MOUNTAIN
NATIONAL/MORMON LOOP TRAIL

DISTANCE: 5 MILES TOTAL
TIME: 3 HOURS OR SO
EFFORT: MEDIUM
(BRING DOUBLE EXTRA WATER)
TYPE: UP & DOWN LOOP
ROUTE SKILL: EASY
(SIGNED ALL THE WAY)
BEST SEASON: OCT to MAY
(CROWDED ON WEEKENDS)
WILDFLOWERS: FEB to APR

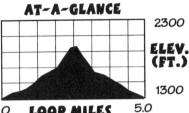

AT-A-GLANCE

2300
ELEV.
(FT.)
1300

0   **LOOP MILES**   5.0

PETS: DOGS ON LEASH

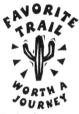

FAVORITE
TRAIL
WORTH A
JOURNEY

DESCRIPTION: One of the most popular hikes and mountain bike rides in Arizona. The gorgeous rugged terrain and superb single track of National/Mormon Loop is legend across the nation among sprocket heads as the "Teacher of Terror". Instead of broken bones and eyes glued to trail, us lucky duck hikers can instead ogle scenery. If the climb does not grab your breath, the views will. Hike all the way up to Buena Vista Lookout if time allows. The Phoenix Mountains Preserve sky islands are in easy view. Sky Harbor, Bank One Ballpark and downtown are at your feet. Pick out Red Mountain, The McDowells and The Superstitions.

MILEAGE LOG

0.0   Begin near the sign at the west end of the parking lot.
1.2   End of the dirt road. National Trail sign is above a wash.
1.3   JUNCTION. National /Mormon Loop splits. Take National.
2.4   REJOIN Mormon. Go RIGHT on Mormon OR up to Buena Vista Lookout if time permits. Hidden Valley Loop is also a great side excursion. See the map.
2.6   RIGHT and down on Mormon Loop Trail.
3.9   Trail returns to Pima Canyon Road.
5.0   Back to GO.

DIRECTIONS: From Phoenix hop on I-10 and head in the DIRECTION of TUCSON. Take BASELINE ROAD EXIT. Go WEST ON BASELINE a few blocks to 48TH STREET. Turn LEFT on 48TH and go just past Guadalupe Road to the PIMA CANYON ROAD park entrance on your RIGHT. Go all the way to the main parking area near the ramadas at the end of the road. Trail heads up dirt road at the west end of the lot.

SOUTH MOUNTAIN
PIMA CANYON TRAILS

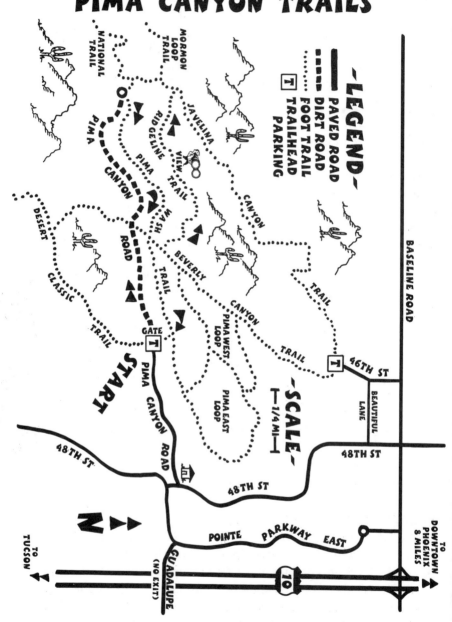

SOUTH MOUNTAIN
PIMA CANYON TRAILS
RIDGELINE/PIMA CANYON WASH LOOP

DISTANCE: 3.1 MILES TOTAL
TIME: 2 HOURS
EFFORT: MODERATE
TYPE: LOOP
ROUTE SKILL: EASY
(SIGNED ALL THE WAY)
BEST SEASON: OCT to MAY
(HIKE AT DAWN IN SUMMER)
WILDFLOWERS: FEB to APR

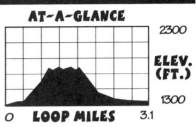

AT-A-GLANCE

2300

ELEV.
(FT.)

1300

0   **LOOP MILES**   3.1

PETS: DOGS ON LEASH

DESCRIPTION: Get above the smog real quick or explore a quiet Sonoran Desert ecosystem. A palo verde tree lined wash is great for early morning birdsong or an encounter with Wily Coyote and Roadrunner. Cacti are abundant as are other hikers and mountain bikers. Find at least 25 miles of trail just in this one tiny area or use it for a launching pad to National/Mormon/Desert Classic Trails in South Mountain's vast trail network. I outline a personal favorite loop that samples the best of what Pima Canyon offers by way of views, plants, reptiles, birds and a darn fine walk.

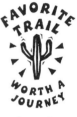

FAVORITE TRAIL — WORTH A JOURNEY

MILEAGE LOG

0.0 Begin near sign and gate at the west end of the parking lot. Head out the dirt road toward tall powerlines.

0.6 RIGHT onto trail at powerline.

0.7 LEFT onto RIDGELINE TRAIL and head UP over four small peaks and the dips in between. Great views then down.

1.6 LEFT at JUNCTION with JAVELINA TRAIL. Go down toward dirt road. Look for brown post in shallow wash near the bottom marking Pima Wash Trail. See map.

1.9 Follow the wash trail down and back to the parking lot.

3.1 A small trail up out of the wash leads to parking area.

DIRECTIONS: From Phoenix hop on I-10 and head in the DIRECTION of TUCSON. Take BASELINE ROAD EXIT. Go WEST ON BASELINE a few blocks to 48TH STREET. Turn LEFT on 48TH and go just past Guadalupe Road to the PIMA CANYON ROAD park entrance on your RIGHT. Go all the way to the main parking area near the ramadas at the end of the road. Trail heads up dirt road at the west end of the lot.

PIMA CANYON TRAILS
SOUTH MTN

SQUAW PEAK (PIESTEWA PEAK)
CIRCUMFERENCE TRAIL #302

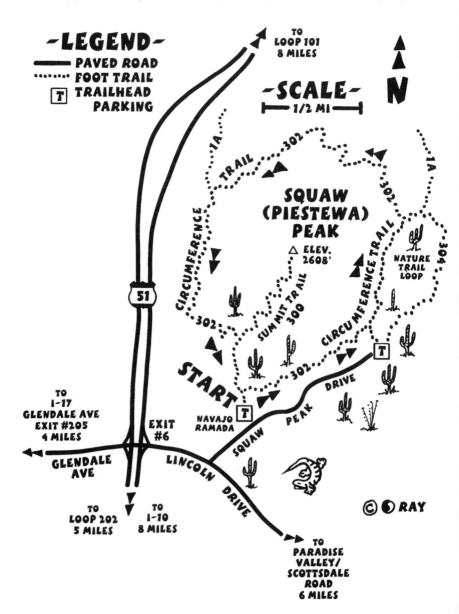

-LEGEND-
— PAVED ROAD
······· FOOT TRAIL
[T] TRAILHEAD PARKING

TO LOOP 101 8 MILES

-SCALE-
1/2 MI

N

SQUAW (PIESTEWA) PEAK
△ ELEV. 2608'

1A
TRAIL
302
1A

CIRCUMFERENCE
302

CIRCUMFERENCE TRAIL
302

NATURE TRAIL LOOP
304

SUMMIT TRAIL 300

51

START

NAVAJO RAMADA
[T]

SQUAW PEAK DRIVE
302

[T]

TO I-17 GLENDALE AVE EXIT #205 4 MILES

EXIT #6

GLENDALE AVE

LINCOLN DRIVE

TO LOOP 202 5 MILES

TO I-10 8 MILES

TO PARADISE VALLEY/ SCOTTSDALE ROAD 6 MILES

© ◗ RAY

SQUAW (PIESTEWA) PEAK
CIRCUMFERENCE TRAIL #302

DISTANCE: 3.7 MILES TOTAL
TIME: AT LEAST 3 HOURS
EFFORT: FAIRLY TOUGH
(THREE GOOD PASSES)
TYPE: LOOP
ROUTE SKILL: EASY
(SIGNED ALL THE WAY)
BEST SEASON: OCT to MAY
(TOO HOT IN DEAD OF SUMMER)
WILDFLOWERS: FEB to APR

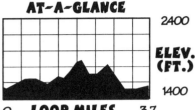

AT-A-GLANCE

2400

ELEV.
(FT.)

1400

0   **LOOP MILES**   3.7

PETS: No dogs on Summit
Trail portion of the loop

DESCRIPTION: Once you've been to the top of the mountain, the next feather in your cap is the tougher loop around Squaw Peak. It's not just a walk through a beautiful, rolling Sonoran Desert ecosystem. Fact is that you will not see one tenth the hoards of Summit Trail. Route finding is still easy. Keep the mountain over your left shoulder. The trail is marked.

Circumference Trail starts off at the Apache Ramada Trailhead at the far end of Squaw Peak Drive just to the left of the information sign. Start down a paved path into a deep wash and scramble up the other side. Now head north up along the wash with Squaw Peak over your left shoulder.

MILEAGE LOG

0.0   START at Apache Ramada just to the left of the info sign. At first you will be on Nature Trail Loop #304.
0.1   JOIN Circumference Trail #302 and continue RIGHT. Go over a low saddle.
0.6   Trail JUNCTION. Take a breather on the bench then go LEFT on #302. Go over another much higher saddle.
1.7   Trail JUNCTION. Go LEFT on #302. Climb again.
2.7   SUMMIT TRAIL #300 JUNCTION. Go RIGHT and DOWN.
3.2   LEFT at the bottom and start heading north again.
3.7   Back to Apache Ramada.

DIRECTIONS: From anywhere in Phoenix, get on the freeway grid and proceed to either LOOP 101 or LOOP 202. Make your way to HIGHWAY 51, Squaw Peak (Piestewa) Freeway. Take the Glendale /Lincoln EXIT #6. Head EAST on Lincoln. After a half mile turn LEFT onto Squaw Peak Drive. Go all the way to the end and park at the Apache Ramada. The trailhead is just to the left of the information sign marked #302/#304.

CIRCUMFERENCE TRAIL
SQUAW PEAK

SQUAW PEAK (PIESTEWA PEAK)
DREAMY DRAW NATURE LOOP

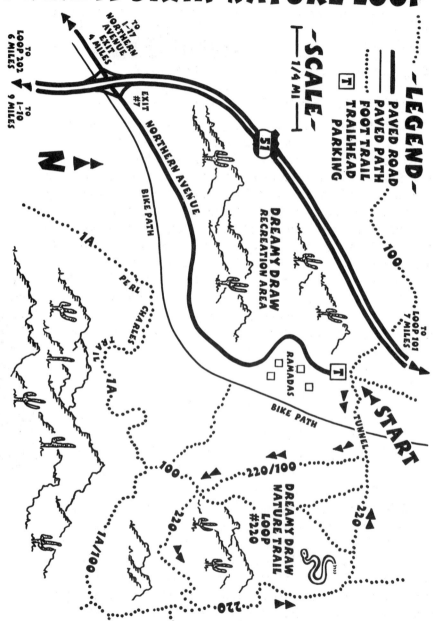

-LEGEND-

PAVED ROAD
PAVED PATH
FOOT TRAIL
T TRAILHEAD PARKING

-SCALE-
1/4 MI

N

TO I-17 NORTHERN AVENUE EXIT 4 MILES
TO LOOP 202 6 MILES
TO I-10 9 MILES

EXIT #7

NORTHERN AVENUE

BIKE PATH

51

100

TO LOOP 101 7 MILES

DREAMY DRAW RECREATION AREA

1A

PERL CHARLES TRAIL

1A

1A/100

RAMADAS

BIKE PATH

T

TUNNEL

START

100

220/100

220

220

DREAMY DRAW NATURE TRAIL LOOP #220

220

SQUAW (PIESTEWA) PEAK
DREAMY DRAW NATURE TRAIL LOOP #220

DISTANCE: 1.5 MILES TOTAL
TIME: 1 HOUR
EFFORT: PRETTY EASY
TYPE: LOOP
ROUTE SKILL: EASY
(SIGNED #220 ALL THE WAY)
BEST SEASON: OCT to MAY
(VERY EARLY MORNINGS IN SUMMER)
WILDFLOWERS: FEB to APR

AT-A-GLANCE

2400

ELEV. (FT.)

1400

O   **LOOP MILES**   1.5

PETS: BRING A LEASH

DESCRIPTION: Scenic, short, easy nature loop trail through Sonoran Desert ecosystem with great views to walk or run when time is short. Fine for pets and kids. Many trails in this area, but hard to get lost so close to the wooshing sound of a busy freeway. Keep an eye out for posts marked #220.

MILEAGE LOG

0.0 Trailhead is at north end of parking lot. Follow up a dry wash and go RIGHT at the "horse tunnel" sign and a trail #220 marker. Continue up the desert-tree lined wash and through the tunnel.

0.2 RIGHT on #220. View Squaw (Piestewa) Peak up ahead.

0.5 JUNCTION with Trail #100. Stay LEFT on #220.

0.7 JUNCTION. Go LEFT and contour around the brushy mountain side. Brittlebush flowers bright yellow in a wet spring burst of color. Saguaros rise up here and there.

0.9 High point. North Mountain's antennas and Lookout Mountain loom ahead. Pinnacle Peak rises northeast. Listen to the steady drone of freeway. Desert is divided, devoured and surrounded daily as every new section of grid connects and closes in. Enjoy the view. Follow the green #220 signs all the way back to the trailhead.

1.5 Back to GO.

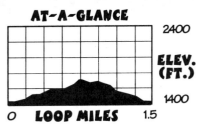

DREAMY DRAW LOOP
SQUAW PEAK

DIRECTIONS: From anywhere in Phoenix, proceed to either LOOP 101 or LOOP 202. See freeway map in centerfold of this book. Make your way to HIGHWAY 51, Squaw Peak (Piestewa) Freeway. Take NORTHERN AVENUE Exit #7 and go EAST into Dreamy Draw Recreation Area and all the way to end of road. Park near the trailhead sign and begin there.

"Shopping is not creating. You are not what you own."
- post modern proverb

SQUAW PEAK
(PIESTEWA PEAK)
MOJAVE TRAIL #200

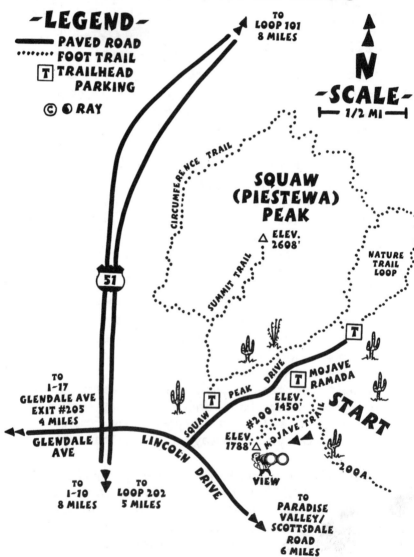

-LEGEND-
- —— PAVED ROAD
- •••••• FOOT TRAIL
- T TRAILHEAD PARKING

© Ⓡ RAY

TO LOOP 101 8 MILES

N

-SCALE-
1/2 MI

CIRCUMFERENCE TRAIL

SQUAW (PIESTEWA) PEAK

△ ELEV. 2608'

SUMMIT TRAIL

NATURE TRAIL LOOP

51

T

MOJAVE RAMADA

T

PEAK DRIVE

SQUAW

TO
I-17
GLENDALE AVE
EXIT #205
4 MILES

T

#200

ELEV. 1450'

ELEV. 1788' △

MOJAVE TRAIL

START

GLENDALE AVE

LINCOLN DRIVE

VIEW

200A

TO
I-10
8 MILES

TO
LOOP 202
5 MILES

TO
PARADISE
VALLEY/
SCOTTSDALE
ROAD
6 MILES

SQUAW (PIESTEWA) PEAK
SHORT MOJAVE TRAIL #200 TO VIEW

DISTANCE: 1 MILE TOTAL
TIME: 1 HOUR
EFFORT: FAIRLY EASY
 (CLIMBS 300 FEET IN HALF-MILE)
TYPE: UP & BACK DOWN
ROUTE SKILL: EASY
 (SIGNED ALL THE WAY)
BEST SEASON: OCT to MAY
WILDFLOWERS: FEB to APR

AT-A-GLANCE

1900

**ELEV.
(FT.)**

1400

O   **1-WAY MILES**   0.5

PETS: DOGS ON LEASH

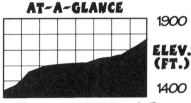

DESCRIPTION: Phoenix Mountains Preserve is a huge open area of rugged Sonoran Desert parkland cutting a diagonal swath right across the heart of Phoenix. The more difficult Summit Trail ascent on Squaw (Piestewa) Peak is a "must do" on the list of every hiker. Hundreds of thousands make that summit pilgrimage every year.

Nearby Mojave Trail on a neighboring hill is shorter, quicker, less arduous and an excellent spot to picnic or sit and enjoy a sunset without so much darn company. The view is no slouch either. With binocs, you can spy on the windows of downtown skyscrapers. As city lights come on, red beacons atop South Mountain define the southern horizon. Planes come and go every minute or two from Sky Harbor. Camelback Mountain is the pyramid to the southeast and best of all, there is a great close up view of Squaw (Piestewa) Peak. Hikers on Summit Trail look like a narrow line of ants.

From the start it is easy to stay found. Just follow Trail #200 markers. Steep at first, after a tenth of a mile the climb mellows out at a junction with Trail #202A. Just stay RIGHT until you reach the rounded summit with plenty of comfortable flat rocks to sit and enjoy.

DIRECTIONS: From anywhere in Phoenix, get on LOOP 101 or LOOP 202. See freeway map in the centerfold of this book. Make your way to HIGHWAY 51, Squaw Peak (Piestewa) Freeway. Take the Glendale Avenue/Lincoln Drive EXIT #6. Now head EAST on Lincoln. After a half mile turn LEFT onto Squaw Peak Drive. Go just another half mile or so and enter the MOJAVE RAMADA on your RIGHT. Park in the highest level of the lot. The trailhead for Mojave Trail #200 is on the right near the lowest ramada next to the information sign.

SQUAW PEAK
(PIESTEWA PEAK)
NATURE LOOP TRAIL #304

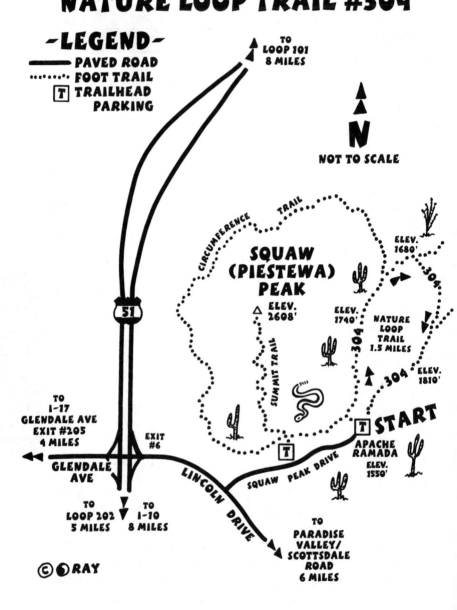

-LEGEND-
━━━ PAVED ROAD
········ FOOT TRAIL
T TRAILHEAD PARKING

TO LOOP 101 8 MILES

N
NOT TO SCALE

CIRCUMFERENCE TRAIL

ELEV. 1680'

SQUAW (PIESTEWA) PEAK
ELEV. 2608'

ELEV. 1740'

304

NATURE LOOP TRAIL 1.5 MILES

304 ELEV. 1810'

SUMMIT TRAIL

51

TO I-17 GLENDALE AVE EXIT #205 4 MILES

EXIT #6

T START
APACHE RAMADA ELEV. 1550'

T

GLENDALE AVE

SQUAW PEAK DRIVE

TO LOOP 202 5 MILES

TO I-10 8 MILES

LINCOLN DRIVE

TO PARADISE VALLEY/ SCOTTSDALE ROAD 6 MILES

© RAY

SQUAW (PIESTEWA) PEAK
NATURE TRAIL LOOP #304

DISTANCE: 1.5 MILES TOTAL
TIME: 1 HOUR
EFFORT: FAIRLY EASY
TYPE: LOOP
ROUTE SKILL: EASY
(SIGNED ALL THE WAY)
BEST SEASON: OCT to MAY
WILDFLOWERS: FEB to APR
(PEAK SEASON MARCH)

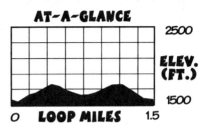

AT-A-GLANCE

2500

**ELEV.
(FT.)**

1500

0   **LOOP MILES**   1.5

PETS: DOGS ON LEASH

DESCRIPTION: Nature Trail #304 is perfect if you want to explore a fairly easy loop trail close to downtown Phoenix in a pristine Sonoran Desert setting. The loop is an interpretive trail with small signs identifying common native plants, so you might just learn a bit about the desert at the same time.

Nature Trail #304 begins as a paved path to the left of the information sign at the north end of the Apache Ramada parking area. Start by descending into a deep wash and back up the other side. Quickly join with Circumference Trail #302 at a junction and continue RIGHT and north along a deep ravine, climbing gradually as Squaw (Piestewa) Peak towers over your left shoulder. Your Sonoran Desert plant education has already begun. The path is lined with saguaro, ocotillo, barrel cactus and, if you arrive following some wet weather, the brilliant yellow flowers of the ubiquitous brittle bush.

You continue over a small saddle then at mile 0.6, the Circumference Trail that winds all the way around Squaw (Piestewa) Peak, takes off to the left. You go RIGHT. This is a good time to sit on the bench provided here and take a pull on your water while checking out the view of the mountain.

Nature Trail next dips into an open area covered with cholla cacti. Careful! Also known as *jumping* cholla. Enough said. Steer clear. Continue over another saddle on well marked #304 until you arrive back at the trailhead.

DIRECTIONS: Easy. From anywhere in Phoenix, get on a freeway and proceed to either LOOP 101 or LOOP 202. See the freeway map in the centerfold of this book. Make your way to HIGHWAY 51, Squaw Peak (Piestewa) Freeway. Take the Glendale Avenue/Lincoln Drive EXIT #6. Now head EAST on Lincoln. After a half mile turn LEFT into Squaw Peak Drive and go all the way to the end. Park near the APACHE RAMADA. The Nature Trail Loop is marked #304.

SQUAW PEAK
(PIESTEWA PEAK)
PERL CHARLES LOOP TRAIL #1A

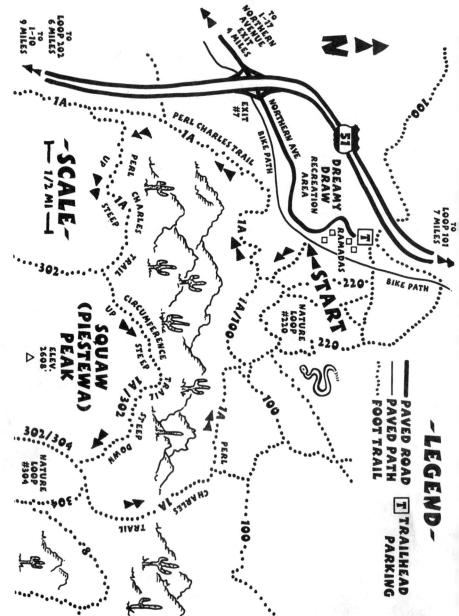

SQUAW (PIESTEWA) PEAK

PERL CHARLES LOOP TRIAL #1A

DISTANCE: 5.9 MILES TOTAL
TIME: 3 HOURS
EFFORT: FAIRLY TOUGH
(ONE STUDLY CLIMB)
TYPE: LOOP
ROUTE SKILL: EASY
(SIGNED 1-A ALL THE WAY)
BEST SEASON: OCT to MAY
(A BIG FAT BUMMER IN SUMMER)
WILDFLOWERS: FEB to APR **PETS:** BRING A LEASH

AT-A-GLANCE

2200

ELEV. (FT.)

1200

0   **LOOP MILES**   5.9

DESCRIPTION: Under bad advice, I did Perl Charles Loop with a mountain bike some years ago. I walked the steep stuff. I remember telling myself at the time, "This ain't no damn ride. This is a hike." Some time later I left the bike home and did just that. And it's a *great* hike, I might add, but still a long way and a grunt to do the big up and over at about the halfway point. Leave your bike home. You'll love it. Lots of giant saguaro, cholla, fish hook barrel cactus, ocotillo and wildflowers aplenty in the spring after a rainy winter. You are in a city of millions and you will likely see not one soul all day.

MILEAGE LOG

0.0 START just east of the parking area above the ramadas. There are many trails in this area. See the map.
0.4 RIGHT at Junction. Trail is now marked "1A" all the way.
1.6 JUNCTION. Go LEFT up and over small saddle.
2.6 JUNCTION with Squaw (Piestewa) Peak Circle Trail 302. LEFT on 1A/302 up and over the steep saddle.
3.8 3-way JUNCTION. Go LEFT on 1A.
5.0 JUNCTION with Trail #100. Stay LEFT and CONTINUE 1A.
5.5 JUNCTION. This is where you came in. Go RIGHT.
5.9 Back to GO.

DIRECTIONS: From anywhere in Phoenix, proceed to either LOOP 101 or LOOP 202. See freeway map in centerfold of this book. Make your way to HIGHWAY 51, Squaw Peak (Piestewa) Freeway. Take NORTHERN AVENUE Exit #7 and go EAST into Dreamy Draw Recreation Area and all the way to end of road. Park near trailhead sign. Begin your hike just east of the parking area above the ramadas. See the map.

"Madness takes its toll. Have exact change ready."
-popular proverb

PERL CHARLES LOOP SQUAW PEAK

SQUAW PEAK (PIESTEWA PEAK)
QUARTZ RIDGE LOOP

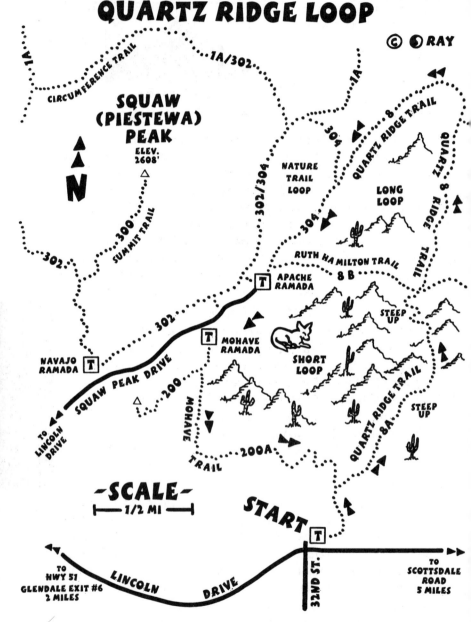

© ☾ RAY

1A

CIRCUMFERENCE TRAIL

1A/302

SQUAW (PIESTEWA) PEAK
ELEV. 2608'

N

302

300

SUMMIT TRAIL

302

302/304

304

1A

8

QUARTZ RIDGE TRAIL

QUARTZ 8 RIDGE TRAIL

NATURE TRAIL LOOP

LONG LOOP

RUTH HAMILTON TRAIL

8 B

STEEP UP

APACHE RAMADA

302

MOHAVE RAMADA

SHORT LOOP

NAVAJO RAMADA

SQUAW PEAK DRIVE

200

MOHAVE TRAIL

QUARTZ RIDGE TRAIL

8A

STEEP UP

TO LINCOLN DRIVE

200A

~SCALE~
1/2 MI

START

T

32ND ST.

TO HWY 51 GLENDALE EXIT #6 2 MILES

LINCOLN DRIVE

TO SCOTTSDALE ROAD 5 MILES

SQUAW (PIESTEWA) PEAK
QUARTZ RIDGE LOOP TRAILS

DISTANCE: 4.6 MILES
(SHORT LOOP 3.4 MILES)
TIME: 3-4 HOURS
EFFORT: MEDIUM TO TOUGH
TYPE: LOOPS
ROUTE SKILL: EASY
(SIGNED ALL THE WAY)
BEST SEASON: OCT to MAY
(HIKE AT DAWN IN SUMMER)
WILDFLOWERS: FEB to APR

AT-A-GLANCE

2400

**ELEV.
(FT.)**

1400

O   **TOTAL MILES**   4.6
(LONG LOOP)

PETS: DOGS ON LEASH

DESCRIPTION: Plenty of geology, flora and fauna just east of busy main Squaw (Piestewa) Peak Trailhead area. Giant saguaro, staghorn, hedgehog, cholla and barrel cacti. Less people mean more animals in this area. Quail, hawk, roadrunner, cactus wren, rabbit, coyote and lots of lizards easily spotted. Stay on trail. Carry lots of water. Do not throw rocks. Avoid Mr. Western Diamondback rattler if lucky enough to see one. Do not approach. This is his home. You are the guest. Long loop takes you out Quartz Ridge Trail #8A, #8 and returns via Mojave Trail #200A. Shortcut across #8B if you go the shorter alternative. All trails are very well marked.

MILEAGE LOG
(LONG LOOP)

0.0 TRAILHEAD. Head out #8A/200A. Lookit da' map.
0.2 JUNCTION. Go RIGHT on #8A. Begin steep ascent.
1.1 SUMMIT then 4-way JUNCTION. Go LEFT for shortcut return on Trail #8B or STRAIGHT on #8 for LONG LOOP.
1.7 JUNCTION. Continue LEFT on #8.
2.4 JUNCTION. Take a LEFT on #304. See the map.
2.8 TRAILHEAD. Walk down paved road to Mojave Trailhead.
3.2 Mojave Trailhead. Find #200A at LEFT of upper ramada.
       #200A goes up, over and contours around to #8A.
4.4 JUNCTION. Go RIGHT on #8A.
4.6 FINISH. You made it!

DIRECTIONS: From HIGHWAY 51, Squaw Peak (Piestewa) Freeway take Glendale Ave. EXIT #6. Go EAST on Lincoln. After a mile and a half turn LEFT on 32nd Street and a quick RIGHT into the trailhead parking. No water or bathrooms here, but there is a shopping center across the street.

QUARTZ RIDGE
SQUAW PEAK

SQUAW PEAK*
(PIESTEWA PEAK)
SUMMIT TRAIL

* TIME FOR A CHANGE. THE WORD "SQUAW" IS A DEMEANING LABEL FOR A NATIVE AMERICAN WOMAN. THE COMBAT DEATH OF SOLDIER LORI PIESTEWA IN 2003 PROVIDED OPPORTUNITY TO RENAME THIS PEAK AND PROVIDE HONOR FOR ALL NATIVE AMERICAN WOMEN. THE CHANGE IS OFFICIAL, BUT OLD SIGNAGE TEMPORARILY REMAINS. TO AVOID CONFUSION I USE BOTH NAMES FOR THE TIME BEING, BUT WILL GREATLY ENJOY HONORING THE CHANGE IN FUTURE EDITIONS.

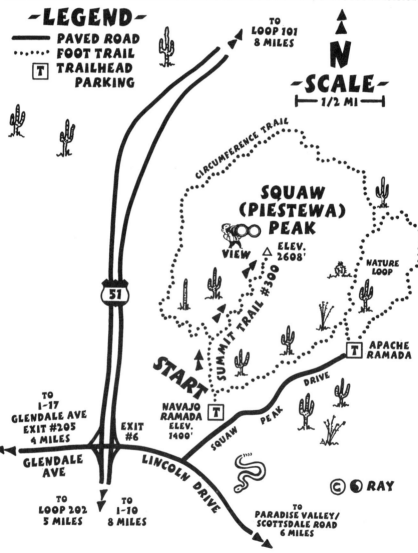

-LEGEND-

—— PAVED ROAD
······ FOOT TRAIL
[T] TRAILHEAD PARKING

N

-SCALE-
⊢ 1/2 MI ⊣

TO
LOOP 101
8 MILES

CIRCUMFERENCE TRAIL

SQUAW (PIESTEWA) PEAK

VIEW
△ ELEV. 2608'

NATURE LOOP

51

SUMMIT TRAIL #300

APACHE RAMADA [T]

START

DRIVE

NAVAJO RAMADA ELEV. 1400' [T]

TO
I-17
GLENDALE AVE
EXIT #205
4 MILES

EXIT #6

SQUAW PEAK

GLENDALE AVE

LINCOLN DRIVE

© ⦿ RAY

TO
LOOP 202
5 MILES

TO
I-10
8 MILES

TO
PARADISE VALLEY/
SCOTTSDALE ROAD
6 MILES

SQUAW (PIESTEWA) PEAK
SUMMIT TRAIL #300 TO PANORAMIC VIEW

DISTANCE: 2.4 MILES TOTAL
TIME: 1.5 TO 2 HOURS
EFFORT: SHORT & STEEP
TYPE: UP & BACK DOWN
ROUTE SKILL: WAY EASY
(SIGNED ALL THE WAY)
BEST SEASON: OCT to MAY
(VERY CROWDED ON WEEKENDS)
WILDFLOWERS: FEB to APR

AT-A-GLANCE

2600

ELEV. (FT.)

1400

O   **1-WAY MILES**   1.2

PETS: NO DOGS ALLOWED

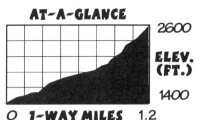

FAVORITE TRAIL

WORTH A JOURNEY

DESCRIPTION: Yikes! They say 500,000 a year summit Squaw (Piestewa) Peak. I believe it. It's a circus on weekends. Some hike the summit for a challenge and the killer views. Some come to get above the brown air or for the great cell phone reception. But most, like me, just come to hike . . . and people watch.

It is *very* steep. It should take at least 45 minutes to an hour for a normal human to summit. Buff, toned and tan types manage to run it in 15 minutes! There is no water or shade, only thirst and work.

There are two summits. 2280' North Summit and 2600' South Summit. Do both for bragging rights to all views. South Mountain's antennas are due south. North Mountain is nearby to the northwest. East set the McDowells, Four Peaks and The Superstitions. Camelback, not looking terribly camel-like from this angle, is nearby to the east-southeast. On a *super* clear day to the southeast you might also spot "Ship of the Desert" Picacho Peak 60 miles distant or the Catalinas near Tucson 100 miles away, but those days are pretty rare.

DIRECTIONS: Easy. From anywhere in Phoenix, get on a freeway and proceed to either LOOP 101 or LOOP 202. See the freeway map in the centerfold of this book. Make your way to HIGHWAY 51, Squaw Peak (Piestewa) Freeway. Take the Glendale Avenue/Lincoln Drive EXIT #6. Now head EAST on Lincoln. After a half mile turn LEFT onto Squaw Peak Drive. Go another half mile and park near the NAVAJO RAMADA on your LEFT. The trailhead for Summit Trail is marked #300.

SUMMIT TRAIL SQUAW PEAK

SUPERSTITION MOUNTAINS
TREASURE LOOP TRAIL
(LOST DUTCHMAN STATE PARK)

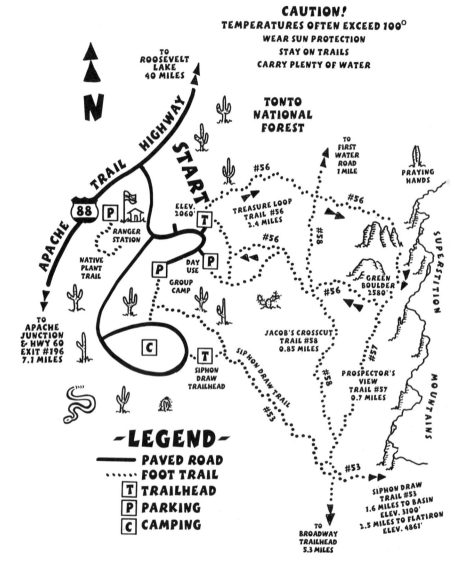

CAUTION!
TEMPERATURES OFTEN EXCEED 100°
WEAR SUN PROTECTION
STAY ON TRAILS
CARRY PLENTY OF WATER

N

TO ROOSEVELT LAKE 40 MILES

TONTO NATIONAL FOREST

TO FIRST WATER ROAD 1 MILE

PRAYING HANDS

APACHE TRAIL HIGHWAY

START

ELEV. 2060'

88

P

RANGER STATION

NATIVE PLANT TRAIL

P DAY USE P

GROUP CAMP

C

T SIPHON DRAW TRAILHEAD

TO APACHE JUNCTION & HWY 60 EXIT #196 7.1 MILES

#56

TREASURE LOOP TRAIL #56 2.4 MILES

#56

#56

#58

GREEN BOULDER 2580'

#56

JACOB'S CROSSCUT TRAIL #58 0.85 MILES

SIPHON DRAW TRAIL

#58

#57

PROSPECTOR'S VIEW TRAIL #57 0.7 MILES

SUPERSTITION MOUNTAINS

#53

#53

TO BROADWAY TRAILHEAD 5.3 MILES

SIPHON DRAW TRAIL #53 1.6 MILES TO BASIN ELEV. 3100' 2.5 MILES TO FLATIRON ELEV. 4861'

~LEGEND~
— PAVED ROAD
····· FOOT TRAIL
T TRAILHEAD
P PARKING
C CAMPING

SUPERSTITION MOUNTAINS
(LOST DUTCHMAN STATE PARK)
THE TREASURE LOOP TRAIL

DISTANCE: 2.5 MILES
TIME: 1.5 to 2 HOURS
EFFORT: EASY to MODERATE
TYPE: SIGNED LOOP
ROUTE SKILL: EASY
(SIGNED ALL THE WAY)
BEST SEASON: OCT to MAY
WILDFLOWERS: FEB to APR
(PEAK SEASON MARCH)

AT-A-GLANCE

3250

ELEV. (FT.)

2000

0   **LOOP MILES**   2.5
(TREASURE LOOP)

DESCRIPTION: Lost Dutchman State Park is named after the legendary 1870s lost gold mine of German Jacob Waltz. He is said to have successfully found and worked a fabulous vein, then stashed one or more caches of gold throughout The Superstitions. Unfortunately for us, Mr. Waltz lacked the courtesy to leave behind a map or coherent description directing us to his booty. Dang, isn't that always the way?!

Treasure Loop is a fairly short, easy and up close look at The Superstitions. The trail is signed and easy to follow. The views are vast. Phoenix skyscrapers look like a Lilliputian Lego-toy town way far away in the distance. Underfoot you get a feel for what lies ahead before you set off into the wilderness seeking fortune on a tougher trail. Safe parking, hiking trails, bathrooms, camping with showers, views and a good information center get you started on the correct foot. Before you leave the info center be sure to check out the quarter-mile Native Plant Trail to familiarize yourself with the selection of prickly flora found throughout these rugged mountains.

Park the car, put the pooch on a leash, grab your hat, bring some water and a snack and begin your hike at the signed Treasure Loop Trailhead located on the north side of the Cholla Day Use Area. It's the first left after leaving the visitor center.

DIRECTIONS: Head EAST out of Phoenix on Superstition Freeway Highway 60 for 25 miles to Apache Junction. Take Idaho Road exit #196. Follow Idaho Road NORTH into Apache Junction for 2.1 miles. You will already see The Superstitions looming overhead. Go RIGHT on Apache Trail, Highway 88 for another 5 miles and turn RIGHT into Lost Dutchman State Park entrance.

TREASURE LOOP TRAIL **SUPERSTITIONS**

SUPERSTITION MOUNTAINS
SIPHON DRAW TRAIL
(LOST DUTCHMAN STATE PARK)

TO ROOSEVELT LAKE 40 MILES

-LEGEND-
— PAVED ROAD
······· FOOT TRAIL
T P TRAILHEAD/ PARKING
C CAMPGROUND

TRAIL HIGHWAY

P
RANGER STATION

APACHE

88

T
P

LOST DUTCHMAN STATE PARK

TO FIRST WATER ROAD

SIPHON DRAW TRAILHEAD ELEV. 2100'

C

CROSSCUT TRAIL

PALMER MINE (CLOSED)

P T

TO APACHE JUNCTION & HWY 60 EXIT #196 7.1 MILES

START

SIPHON

JACOB'S

DRAW

THE FLATIRON ELEV. 4861'

SUPERSTITION

N

TRAIL

BOX CANYON TURN AROUND ELEV. 3130'

-SCALE-
⊢ 1/2 MI ⊣

TO BROADWAY TRAILHEAD 5.3 MILES

THE CRYING DINOSAUR

MOUNTAINS

SUPERSTITION MOUNTAINS
(LOST DUTCHMAN STATE PARK)
SIPHON DRAW TRAIL #53

DISTANCE: 3.2 MILES TOTAL
TIME: 2.5 to 3 HOURS
EFFORT: EASY to MODERATE
TYPE: OUT & BACK
ROUTE SKILL: EASY
BEST SEASON: OCT to MAY
WILDFLOWERS: FEB to APR
(PEAK SEASON MARCH)

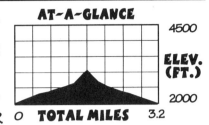

AT-A-GLANCE

ELEV. (FT.)
4500
2000

O   **TOTAL MILES**   3.2

DESCRIPTION: Views of The Superstition's sheer cliffs and wild peaks tower above Lost Dutchman State Park. A fairly easy canyon hike cuts into the face of this impenetrable and forbidding wall of stone. In spring, the path is carpeted with yellow brittlebush flowers, but only after we get a good spell of winter rain. Along the way, the abandoned 1886 Palmer Mine is an interesting spot to poke around. After the mine, the trail and canyon narrow as you ascend up through cliffs broken into fantastic shapes. On your right, you'll not squint nor use much imagination to make out The Crying Dinosaur. You'll spot the head, mouth, neck and a crack appearing to be an enormous tear. Boo-hoo. Siphon Draw further narrows and steepens as you continue ever up. The trail crosses a rocky wash before finally ending on the floor of a sheer box canyon under a normally dry waterfall, a good spot to groove on the view and enjoy some snackage before you turn around. Siphon Draw's out-and-back nature make it hard to get lost and easy to return at any point along the way.

If you are somewhat more hard core, you can clamber, climb and bushwhack further up the dry streambed, over boulders and through brush to the top of The Flatiron. This adds 1.8 very steep and tough total miles plus at least 2 more hours to your hike, but the view from the top is pretty dang impressive. A very tough, worthy goal at 4861'.

DIRECTIONS: Head EAST out of Phoenix on Superstition Freeway Highway 60 for 25 miles to Apache Junction. Take Idaho Road exit #196. Follow Idaho Road NORTH into Apache Junction for 2.1 miles. You will plainly see The Superstitions looming overhead. Go RIGHT on Apache Trail, Highway 88 for another 5 miles and turn RIGHT into the Lost Dutchman State Park entrance. The Siphon Draw Trailhead is at the east end of the main campground loop.

SUPERSTITIONS
SIPHON DRAW TRAIL

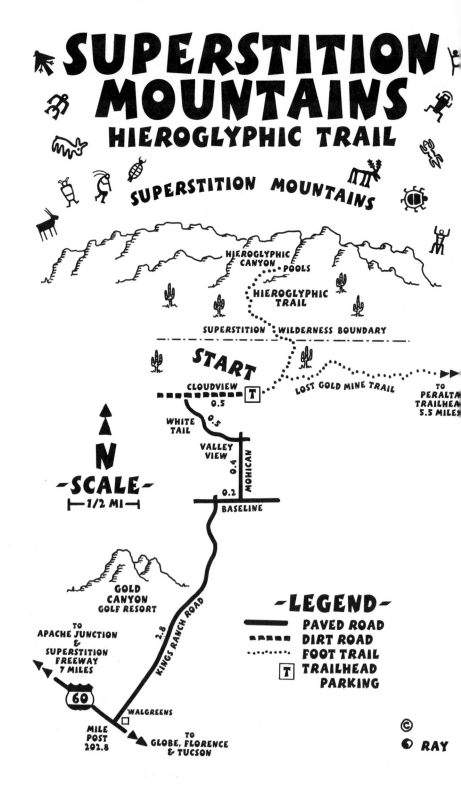

SUPERSTITION MOUNTAINS
HIEROGLYPHIC TRAIL TO PETROGLYPHS

DISTANCE: 4 MILES TOTAL
TIME: 2 to 3 HOURS
EFFORT: FAIRLY EASY
(STEEP AT FIRST, THEN MELLOW)
TYPE: OUT & BACK
ROUTE SKILL: VERY EASY
(SIGNED ALL THE WAY)
BEST SEASON: OCT to MAY
(TOO DARN HOT IN MID-SUMMER)
WILDFLOWERS: FEB to APR

AT-A-GLANCE

3000

**ELEV.
(FT.)**

2000

0   **1-WAY MILES**   2

PETS: DOGS ON LEASH

DESCRIPTION: "Hieroglyphic" is a misnomer. Hohokam petroglyphs date back over 1,000 years, well before European settlement. The art still has that magic connection to the ancient dream world of cave drawings and hunting with spears that existed before recorded time. Very cool.

FAVORITE TRAIL WORTH A JOURNEY

Views are excellent to the east, south and smoggy west (. . . but it's a *dry* smog!) toward Phoenix. Excellent cactus selection. Spot superb saguaro specimens as well as several cholla varieties, hedgehog, prickly pear and ocotillo. Brilliant flowers all along the way. Greenery and water at Hieroglyphic Pools after some wet weather, dry at other times. South facing, sunny and warm all day.

START at parking lot at east end of Cloudview Road. See map. The trail heads up steep at first, but the climb quickly mellows out. After a quarter mile or so the trail splits. A good sign points the way NORTH to Hieroglyphic Canyon.

IMPORTANT NOTES: DO NOT TOUCH THE ART! Many hands over time do damage. This is a popular trail. The nearby area continues to be developed with houses, shops and golf resorts. Please protect our trail access. Obey all private property and no parking signs. Obey the speed limit in the nearby neighborhood. Children and pets present.

DIRECTIONS: From Phoenix head out Superstition Freeway HWY 60 east toward Apache Junction. Continue as freeway ends and go another 7 miles on HWY 60 to milepost 202.8. Go LEFT onto paved Kings Ranch Road heading NORTH. Follow the map to the turnaround/parking area at the end of Cloudview Road. No bathrooms or water at trailhead.

HIEROGLYPHIC TRAIL
SUPERSTITIONS

SUPERSTITION MOUNTAINS
PERALTA CANYON TRAIL

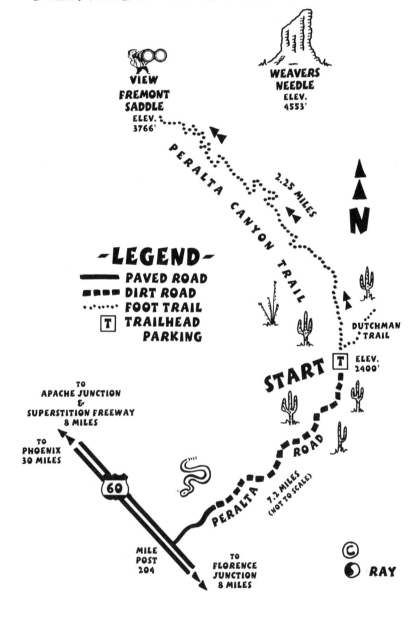

VIEW
FREMONT SADDLE
ELEV. 3766'

WEAVERS NEEDLE
ELEV. 4553'

PERALTA CANYON TRAIL

2.25 MILES

N

-LEGEND-
——— PAVED ROAD
▪▪▪▪ DIRT ROAD
········ FOOT TRAIL
T TRAILHEAD PARKING

DUTCHMAN TRAIL

START

T ELEV. 2400'

TO APACHE JUNCTION & SUPERSTITION FREEWAY 8 MILES

TO PHOENIX 30 MILES

PERALTA ROAD

7.2 MILES (NOT TO SCALE)

60

MILE POST 204

TO FLORENCE JUNCTION 8 MILES

© RAY

SUPERSTITION MOUNTAINS
PERALTA CANYON TRAIL TO SADDLE VIEW

DISTANCE: 4.5 MILES TOTAL
TIME: 3 HOURS
EFFORT: MODERATE
TYPE: UP & BACK DOWN
ROUTE SKILL: EASY
BEST SEASON: OCT to MAY
(CROWDED ON WEEKENDS)
WILDFLOWERS: FEB to APR

AT-A-GLANCE

4000

ELEV. (FT.)

2000

O **1-WAY MILES** 2.25

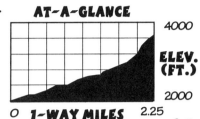

FAVORITE TRAIL
WORTH A JOURNEY

DESCRIPTION: One of the very best hikes in Arizona. If you can do just one trail in The Superstitions, this is it. Monuments, spires, hoodoos, windows, needles, balancing rocks, lizards, wizards, ghouls and goblins . . . all enroute up to Fremont Saddle. From there, get a good look deep into The Superstitions plus a great view of Weaver's Needle, a volcanic plug indicative of the fiery origins of these fabled mountains. For a real close-up of the monument, follow the ridgeline from Fremont Saddle northeast about a quarter mile out to the view spot just opposite Weavers Needle.

Peralta Trail to Fremont Saddle ascends 1366' in 2.25 miles. Figure 2 hours for the climb and 1 hour for the descent. The climb is constant, yet rarely gets steep. Take time to look at the fantastic formations as you go up. There are views aplenty every step of the way. Well worn and easy to follow, the trail is still rough. Do all your looking as you climb. Trail gremlins command your visual attention as your feet gather speed on the way down. A twisted ankle will ruin your day.

Bring lunch for the view spot and don't forget water, a half gallon per person in cool weather and twice that if it's warm out. Thirsty hikers make stupid mistakes.

DIRECTIONS: From Phoenix head out Superstition Freeway HWY 60 east toward Apache Junction. Continue as freeway ends and go another 8 miles on HWY 60 to milepost 204. Go LEFT onto Peralta Road heading north. After a paved mile the road turns washboard dirt, but any car can make it. Keep your speed down as there are some blind corners. Go 7.2 miles to the end of the road, pay your fee and park. This is a very busy trailhead, so leave goodies out of sight or take them with you as there may be thieves about. There are bathrooms at the trailhead, but no water.

PERALTA CANYON TRAIL
SUPERSTITIONS

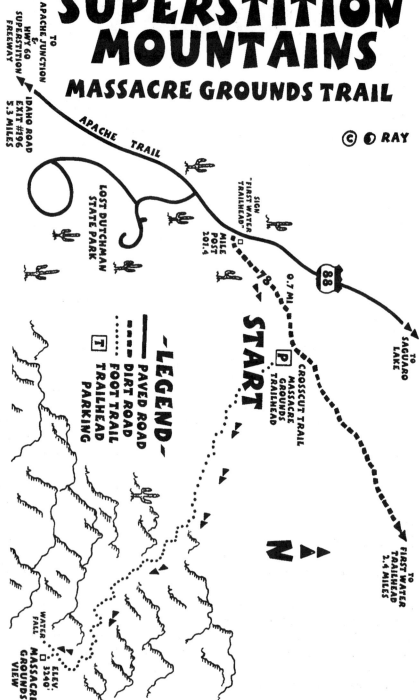

SUPERSTITION MOUNTAINS
MASSACRE GROUNDS TRAIL

© ⊙ RAY

TO
APACHE JUNCTION
&
SUPERSTITION
FREEWAY

HWY 60
SUPERSTITION
FREEWAY

IDAHO ROAD
EXIT #196
5.3 MILES

APACHE TRAIL

LOST DUTCHMAN
STATE PARK

SIGN
"FIRST WATER
TRAILHEAD"

MILE
POST
201.4

78

0.7 MI.

88

TO
SAGUARO
LAKE

START

P MASSACRE
GROUNDS
TRAILHEAD

CROSSCUT TRAIL

N

TO
FIRST WATER
TRAILHEAD
2.4 MILES

-LEGEND-
—— PAVED ROAD
– – – DIRT ROAD
· · · · FOOT TRAIL
T TRAILHEAD PARKING

WATER
FALL

ELEV.
3240'
MASSACRE
GROUNDS
VIEW

SUPERSTITION MOUNTAINS
MASSACRE GROUNDS TRAIL

DISTANCE: 5.2 MILES TOTAL
TIME: 3 HOURS
EFFORT: MEDIUM
(EASY WALK TO STEEP UP)
TYPE: OUT & BACK
ROUTE SKILL: MODERATE
(SIGNED BUT SOME SKILL NEEDED)
BEST SEASON: OCT to MAY
(TOO DANG HOT IN MID-SUMMER)
WILDFLOWERS: FEB to APR

AT-A-GLANCE

3300

ELEV.
(FT.)

2300

O   **1-WAY MILES**   1.5
PETS: DOGS ON LEASH

DESCRIPTION: The Superstition Mountains are richly steeped in history. Some of that history has been dipped in blood. Mexican miners and local Apache had not been getting along. Things came to a head in 1848 when the miners were attempting to remove an amount of gold. The Apaches pinned them down against a rock wall and the Mexican miners died there at a place that came to be know as Massacre Grounds. Once again, gold and blood soaked the soil.

After a wet winter, that blood and gold gives rise to an unimaginable variety of wildflowers. Dozens of species thrive here. Thick and rich carpets of globemallow, poppies, lupine and brittlebush line the trail. When the trail ends at Massacre Grounds, enjoy the vast views in every direction and particularly notice the the black wall against which the miners died. After some quick reflection and a spot of lunch, return the way you came.

The hike to this historic spot is fairly steep, but also fairly short. You climb about 900 feet in 1.5 miles. The trail is uncrowded. You will most likely see nobody. There is no water. Tank up and buy snacks before you leave Apache Junction.

DIRECTIONS: From Phoenix, head EAST on HWY 60, Superstition Freeway, to Apache Junction. Take Idaho Road Exit #196. Go LEFT and NORTH on Idaho Road as it becomes HWY 88, Apache Trail. Continue 5.5 miles to signed First Water Trailhead Road, Forest Service Road 78, at milepost 201.4. Turn RIGHT and continue on smooth dirt road FS 78 for 0.7 miles. Park at the Crosscut Trailhead parking lot. There you will see the signs for Massacre Grounds and Crosscut Trails. There may be a few false spur trails to avoid. Just stay on the main trail and watch for cairns. Check out Massacre Falls during rainy season. See the map.

MASSACRE GROUNDS TRAIL
SUPERSTITIONS

USERY MOUNTAINS
CAT PEAKS LOOP TRAIL

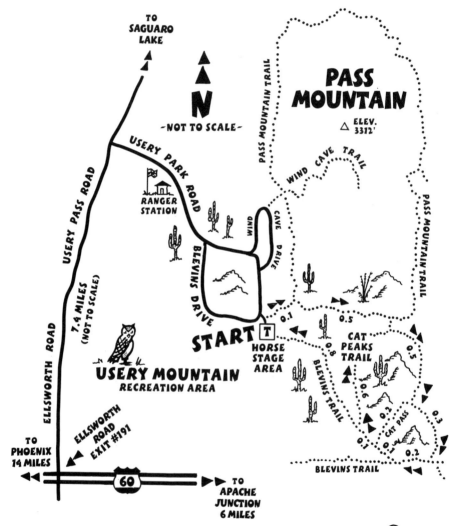

TO SAGUARO LAKE

N
-NOT TO SCALE-

PASS MOUNTAIN TRAIL

PASS MOUNTAIN
△ ELEV. 3312'

USERY PARK ROAD

USERY PASS ROAD

WIND CAVE TRAIL

RANGER STATION

PASS MOUNTAIN TRAIL

7.4 MILES (NOT TO SCALE)

BLEVINS DRIVE

WIND CAVE DRIVE

0.1   0.5

START T
HORSE STAGE AREA

CAT PEAKS TRAIL

0.8   0.5

ELLSWORTH ROAD

USERY MOUNTAIN
RECREATION AREA

BLEVINS TRAIL

0.6   0.2

CAT PASS   0.3

0.1   0.2

TO PHOENIX 14 MILES

ELLSWORTH ROAD EXIT #191

BLEVINS TRAIL

60

TO APACHE JUNCTION 6 MILES

 RAY

USERY MOUNTAIN PARK
CAT PEAKS LOOP TRAIL

DISTANCE: 3 MILES TOTAL
TIME: 1.5 TO 2 HOURS
EFFORT: EASY
(CROSSES A FEW WASHES)
TYPE: LOOP
ROUTE SKILL: EASY
(SIGNED ALL THE WAY)
BEST SEASON: OCT to MAY
WILDFLOWERS: FEB to APR
(SIGNED ALL THE WAY)

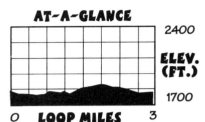

AT-A-GLANCE

2400

**ELEV.
(FT.)**

1700

0   **LOOP MILES**   3

PETS: DOGS ON LEASH

DESCRIPTION: Cat Peaks are named for mountain lion living here once upon a time. Excellent clear view of Superstition Mountains just a few miles to the east. Pass Mountain looms overhead NORTH making for great landmark.

Chances of seeing lion are slim, but because of nearby Tonto National Forest wilderness, you may see bobcat, javelina, coyote, deer, rabbit, species of birds (i.e. owl, hawk, roadrunner, cactus wren and more), reptiles and maybe even a nocturnal ring-tailed cat. Looks like a cute cross between its raccoon cousin and a lemur with enormous bushy ringed tail.

Also, this is a great area for wildflowers after a rainy winter. Bright yellow brittlebush, Mexican gold poppies and purple blue lupine dot the landscape. Many fine examples of cactus as well, especially a few monstrous chain fruit cholla.

MILEAGE LOG

0.0 Leave Horse Stage Area on Pass Mountain Trail. RIGHT at junction and continue to Cat Peaks Trail. See map.
0.6 RIGHT onto Cat Peaks Trail. Loop clockwise.
1.1 JUNCTION with Cat Pass Trail. Good views on top or CONTINUE around Cat Peaks.
1.7 jUNCTION again with the other end of Cat Pass Trail.
1.8 Trail SPLITS. You can return the way you came or return on Blevins Trail.
3.0 Back to Start

DIRECTIONS: From Phoenix go east on the Superstition Freeway, U.S. Highway 60, toward Apache Junction. Take Exit #191, Ellsworth Road. Go LEFT on Ellsworth heading north and continue as Ellsworth Road becomes Usery Pass Road. Go 7.2 miles to park entrance on your right. Stop at ranger station and pay fee. Continue to horse stage area on Blevins Drive. See the map.

USERY MOUNTAINS
MERKL LOOP TRAIL

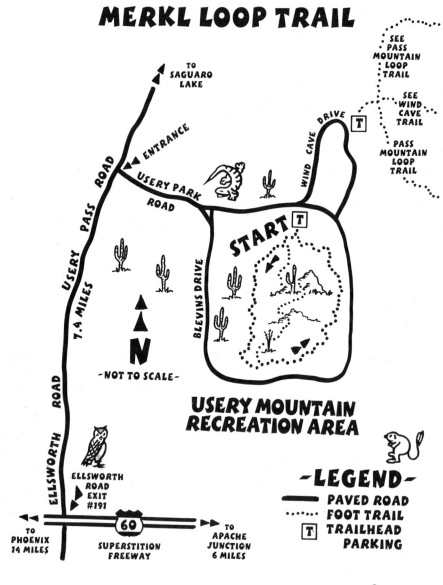

SEE PASS MOUNTAIN LOOP TRAIL

SEE WIND CAVE TRAIL

PASS MOUNTAIN LOOP TRAIL

TO SAGUARO LAKE

ENTRANCE

USERY PARK ROAD

WIND CAVE DRIVE

USERY PASS ROAD

7.4 MILES

BLEVINS DRIVE

START

N

—NOT TO SCALE—

USERY MOUNTAIN RECREATION AREA

ELLSWORTH ROAD

ELLSWORTH ROAD EXIT #191

60

SUPERSTITION FREEWAY

TO PHOENIX 14 MILES

TO APACHE JUNCTION 6 MILES

—LEGEND—
— PAVED ROAD
...... FOOT TRAIL
T TRAILHEAD PARKING

© RAY

USERY MOUNTAIN PARK
MERKL MEMORIAL LOOP TRAIL #140

DISTANCE: 0.9 MILES TOTAL
TIME: 1 HOUR
EFFORT: NO SWEAT
TYPE: LOOP
ROUTE SKILL: EASY
  (SIGNED ALL THE WAY)
BEST SEASON: OCT to MAY
WILDFLOWERS: FEB to APR
  (PEAK SEASON MARCH AND APRIL)

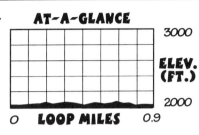

AT-A-GLANCE

3000

ELEV. (FT.)

2000

0   LOOP MILES   0.9

DESCRIPTION: Merkl Loop Trail is short, easy and contains a world of life and beauty for the desert plant lover. Most favorite types of Sonoran Desert cacti can be found along this signed interpretive path . . . saguaro, fishhook barrel, cholla and pincushion to name a few. Springtime incites a neon riot of yellow, purple, red and pink flowers. The skeletal sticks of the ocotillo burst with bright green leaves and topped with even brighter red blooms. Look for baby saguaro in the shade of protective palo verde trees. A saguaro that may reach 30 feet in 150 years may be half the size of your pinky finger. Never tread off trail in this fragile environment.

After the rains of the southwestern desert winter have gone and spring sun warms plants to bloom, Merkl Loop is a feast for the eyeballs. Everywhere flowers carpet the rocky soil along your path. The ubiquitous brittlebush flower is tiny, bright and yellow. Fiddleneck, bursage and popcorn flower surround you. I particularly like the Mexican gold poppy found here and there along the loop. Ephedra, also called Mormon tea, was a favorite drink of early settlers to these parts. I still brew it up from time to time. Tasty and good for what ails ya. Don't pick it though. It's available from your herbalist.

Begin your stroll from the trailhead parking area on Usery Park Road just past Wind Cave Drive. You will find bathrooms, ramadas, a picnic area, water and even a soda machine if memory serves. I like to take the left fork and hike Merkl Loop in a clockwise direction beginning with a great view of The Superstition Mountains looming to the east.

DIRECTIONS: From Phoenix go east on the Superstition Freeway, U.S. Highway 60, toward Apache Junction. Take Exit #191, Ellsworth Road. Go LEFT on Ellsworth heading north and continue as Ellsworth Road becomes Usery Pass Road. Go 7.2 miles to the park entrance on your right.

MERKL LOOP TRAIL
USERY MTNS

USERY MOUNTAINS
PASS MOUNTAIN LOOP TRAIL

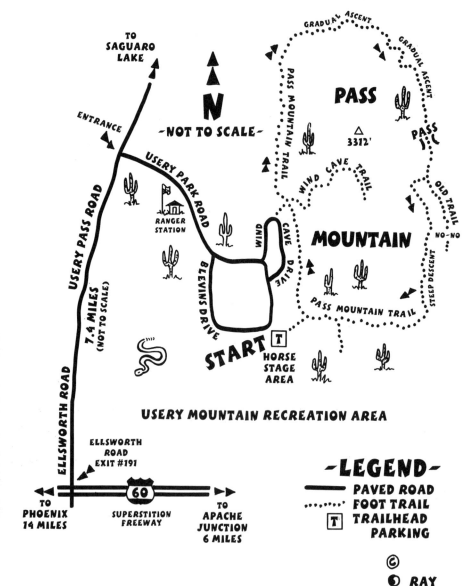

TO SAGUARO LAKE

ENTRANCE

N
~NOT TO SCALE~

USERY PARK ROAD

USERY PASS ROAD

RANGER STATION

BLEVINS DRIVE

7.4 MILES (NOT TO SCALE)

ELLSWORTH ROAD

PASS MOUNTAIN TRAIL

GRADUAL ASCENT

GRADUAL ASCENT

PASS

△ 3312'

PASS

WIND CAVE TRAIL

WIND CAVE DRIVE

MOUNTAIN

OLD TRAIL

NO-NO

STEEP DESCENT

PASS MOUNTAIN TRAIL

START T
HORSE STAGE AREA

USERY MOUNTAIN RECREATION AREA

ELLSWORTH ROAD EXIT #191

60

TO PHOENIX 14 MILES

SUPERSTITION FREEWAY

TO APACHE JUNCTION 6 MILES

-**LEGEND**-
—— PAVED ROAD
········ FOOT TRAIL
T TRAILHEAD PARKING

© RAY

USERY MOUNTAIN PARK
PASS MOUNTAIN LOOP TRAIL

DISTANCE: 7.8 MILES TOTAL
TIME: 3 HOURS
EFFORT: MEDIUM TO TOUGH
(CROSSES SEVERAL WASHES)
TYPE: LOOP
ROUTE SKILL: MODERATE
(PAY ATTENTION TO SIGNS)
BEST SEASON: OCT to APR
WILDFLOWERS: FEB to APR

AT~A~GLANCE

4000

ELEV. (FT.)

1500

O   **LOOP MILES**   7.8

DESCRIPTION: A challenging, rewarding loop around Pass Mountain through pristine Sonoran Desert. Cacti and wild flowers explode in riotous color long about March, but any time in the cooler months is perfect. Too dang hot in summer. You will cross several washes to make you sweat. Around the back side of the mountain the views expand forever, but you don't see any sign of so called civilization. Wear sturdy shoes. Bring lots of water and a snack. Be smart. Go clockwise to climb the loop nice and gradual and then descend steeply.

MILEAGE LOG

0.0 Begin at the horse stage area. See the map. Head east on Pass Mountain Trail. After about 0.2 miles you come to a "T" junction. Go left and you are on the loop.

0.7 Pass Mountain Loop crosses Wind Cave Trail. Go around the north side of the mountain. Cross several washes and you are in wild country. Spy Four Peaks. Go up, up, up. Look around. Great views. No sign of roads, buildings, cars, people, etc. No nothing. Just scenery. Fabulous!

4.4 The Pass. High point of the loop. Begin descent. Trail gets rough at first then better.

4.6 Old trail goes left. You stay RIGHT.

6.1 Unsigned trail junction. Stay RIGHT.

7.1 Cat Peaks Trail junction. Stay RIGHT.

7.6 Back to the "T" junction where you began. Go LEFT.

7.7 Horse stage area.

DIRECTIONS: From Phoenix go east on the Superstition Freeway, U.S. Highway 60, toward Apache Junction. Take Exit #191, Ellsworth Road. Go LEFT on Ellsworth heading north and continue as Ellsworth Road becomes Usery Pass Road. Go 7.2 miles to park entrance on your right.

"If you do not go, you will never know."
- The Buddha

PASS MOUNTAIN LOOP
USERY MTNS

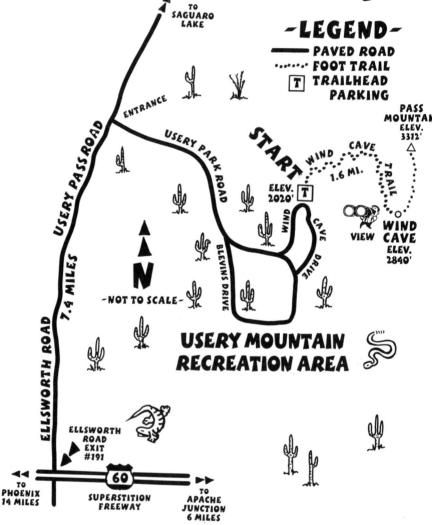

USERY MOUNTAINS
WIND CAVE TRAIL

-LEGEND-

━━━ PAVED ROAD
······ FOOT TRAIL
T TRAILHEAD PARKING

TO SAGUARO LAKE

ENTRANCE

USERY PASS ROAD

USERY PARK ROAD

START

WIND CAVE TRAIL 1.6 MI.

PASS MOUNTAIN ELEV. 3312'

ELEV. 2020' T

WIND CAVE DRIVE

BLEVINS DRIVE

VIEW

WIND CAVE ELEV. 2840'

▲ N

-NOT TO SCALE-

USERY MOUNTAIN RECREATION AREA

7.4 MILES

ELLSWORTH ROAD

ELLSWORTH ROAD EXIT #191

60 SUPERSTITION FREEWAY

◄◄ TO PHOENIX 14 MILES

TO APACHE JUNCTION 6 MILES

©

🌑 RAY

USERY MOUNTAIN PARK
WIND CAVE TRAIL

DISTANCE: 3.2 MILES TOTAL
TIME: 2 HOURS
EFFORT: SHORT & STEEP
(CLIMBS 820 FEET IN 1.6 MILES)
TYPE: OUT & BACK
ROUTE SKILL: EASY
(SIGNED ALL THE WAY)
BEST SEASON: OCT to APR
WILDFLOWERS: FEB to APR
(PEAK SEASON MARCH)

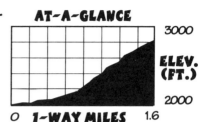

AT~A~GLANCE

3000

ELEV. (FT.)

2000

O **1~WAY MILES** 1.6

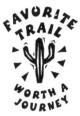

FAVORITE TRAIL

WORTH A JOURNEY

DESCRIPTION: Usery Mountain Recreation Area is located at the base of Pass Mountain covering 3,000 acres and adjoins tens of thousands more in the Tonto National Forest. At the very eastern edge of ever expanding Phoenix metro, the park is prelude to the Superstition Mountains just north and east of Apache Junction.

Wind Cave is a large, northwest facing alcove near the top of Pass Mountain. Shady and damp, water seeps into the roof of the cave supporting lush colonies of flowering vines in the cooler months. The shade provides a welcome respite from relentless sun and a great spot to sit and ponder. Views to the west are epic. The plein aire view of The Valley of the Sun, its sky island peaks and distant tinker-toy town Phoenix will inspire an appetite. Hope you brought snackage.

MILEAGE LOG

0.0 Take off from the trailhead at the north end of Wind Cave Drive. See map. The first bit heads north through the saguaro and brittlebush gradually ascending the plain or *bajada* at the base of Pass Mountain.

0.5 Pull up a rock and catch your breath and a view before heading up. As you approach the cliffs, the trail begins to switch back and get noticeably steeper.

1.6 Wind Cave. Spend some time before going down or look for the 0.4 mile trail option from here to a killer 360° view at the top of Pass Mountain.

3.2 Return to Wind Cave Trailhead.

DIRECTIONS: From Phoenix go east on the Superstition Freeway, U.S. Highway 60, toward Apache Junction. Take Exit #191, Ellsworth Road. Go LEFT on Ellsworth heading north and continue as Ellsworth Road becomes Usery Pass Road. Go 7.2 miles to the park entrance on your right.

WHITE TANK MOUNTAINS
BLACK ROCK (ART) LOOP TRAIL

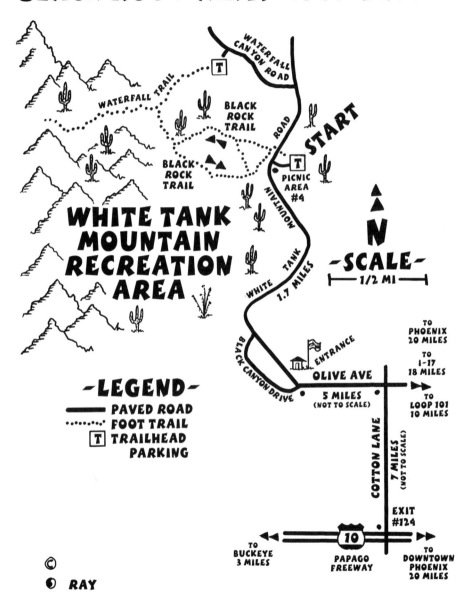

WATERFALL CANYON ROAD

WATERFALL TRAIL

BLACK ROCK TRAIL

ROAD

START

BLACK ROCK TRAIL

T PICNIC AREA #4

MOUNTAIN

WHITE TANK

1.7 MILES

WHITE TANK MOUNTAIN RECREATION AREA

N

~SCALE~
1/2 MI

BLACK CANYON DRIVE

ENTRANCE

OLIVE AVE

TO PHOENIX 20 MILES

TO I-17 18 MILES

TO LOOP 101 10 MILES

5 MILES (NOT TO SCALE)

COTTON LANE

7 MILES (NOT TO SCALE)

EXIT #124

~LEGEND~
— PAVED ROAD
······· FOOT TRAIL
T TRAILHEAD PARKING

10

TO BUCKEYE 3 MILES

PAPAGO FREEWAY

TO DOWNTOWN PHOENIX 20 MILES

© RAY

DISTANCE: 1.8 MILE LOOP
(1.1 MILE SHORT LOOP)

TIME: 1 HOUR

EFFORT: VERY EASY

TYPE: LONG OR SHORT LOOP

ROUTE SKILL: EASY
(SIGNED ALL THE WAY)

BEST SEASON: OCT to MAY
(HIKE VERY VERY EARLY IN SUMMER)

WILDFLOWERS: FEB to APR **PETS:** DOGS ON LEASH

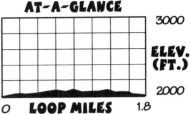

AT-A-GLANCE

3000

ELEV. (FT.)

2000

0   **LOOP MILES**   1.8
(LONG LOOP)

DESCRIPTION: Excellent Hohokam rock art. Two fairly flat loops. Perfect for kids. Short loop is wheelchair friendly. Interpretive displays along the way illustrate information about geology, plants, animals and ancient petroglyphs.

The White Tanks define the horizon west of Phoenix. Sudden, heavy summer rain gushes from canyons forming pools or tanks. Water attracts animals. Animals attract hunters. Dark desert varnish that forms on white granite was perfect for ancient hunters to scribe their wily visions. Be wily yourself, carry adequate water and stay on the trail.

MILEAGE LOG
(LONG LOOP)

0.0 START at trailhead at northwest side of parking lot. Trail crosses the main park road. Watch for cars. Trail splits. Go RIGHT and loop counter-clockwise.

0.4 Look up on boulders to your LEFT. Petroglyphs.

0.5 SIGNED JUNCTION. Decision time. Short, barrier-free loop goes LEFT. Longer loop continues RIGHT.

0.8 JUNCTION with shortcut to Waterfall Trail. See map.

1.1 Excellent petroglyphs etched on boulders above trail on the RIGHT.

1.3 JUNCTION. Trail rejoins with short loop.

1.8 Easy walk back to GO.

DIRECTIONS: From Phoenix take I-10 west for 20 miles to Cotton Lane Exit #124. Go RIGHT and head NORTH 7 miles on Cotton to Olive Avenue and turn LEFT. Go another 5 miles to park entrance. Pick up one of the new superb FREE park topo maps then CONTINUE about 1.7 miles to group picnic area #4 on the RIGHT. Park in the lot.

BLACK ROCK LOOP TRAIL
WHITE TANKS

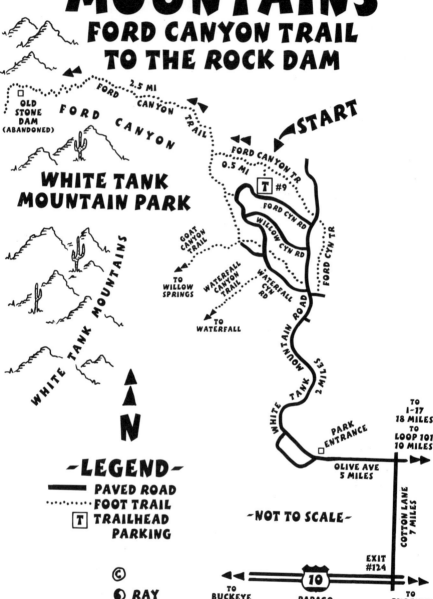

WHITE TANK MOUNTAINS

FORD CANYON TRAIL
TO THE ROCK DAM

OLD STONE DAM (ABANDONED)

FORD CANYON

2.5 MI
FORD CANYON TRAIL

START

FORD CANYON TR

0.5 MI

T #9

FORD CYN RD

WILLOW CYN RD

FORD CYN TR

WHITE TANK MOUNTAIN PARK

GOAT CANYON TRAIL

TO WILLOW SPRINGS

WATERFALL CANYON TRAIL

WATERFALL CYN RD

TO WATERFALL

WHITE TANK MOUNTAINS

WHITE TANK MOUNTAIN ROAD

2 MILES

N

PARK ENTRANCE

TO I-17 18 MILES
TO LOOP 101 10 MILES

OLIVE AVE 5 MILES

COTTON LANE 7 MILES

-LEGEND-

—— PAVED ROAD
·········· FOOT TRAIL
T TRAILHEAD PARKING

-NOT TO SCALE-

EXIT #124

© RAY

10

TO BUCKEYE 3 MILES

PAPAGO FREEWAY

TO PHOENIX 20 MILES

WHITE TANK MOUNTAINS
FORD CANYON TRAIL TO OLD ROCK DAM

DISTANCE: 6 MILES TOTAL
TIME: 3 HOURS
EFFORT: MOSTLY EASY
(GETS TOUGHER AT THE VERY END)
TYPE: OUT & BACK
ROUTE SKILL: EASY
(SIGNED ALL THE WAY)
BEST SEASON: OCT to MAY
WILDFLOWERS: FEB to APR
(PEAK SEASON MARCH)
PETS: DOGS ON LEASH

AT~A~GLANCE

2000

ELEV.
(FT.)

1500

0   **1~WAY MILES**   3.0

DESCRIPTION: Ford Canyon drains a big section of the White Tank Mountains onto a wide bajada or plain at the foot of The White Tanks. Swift rainwater passing over the bajada encourages abundant wildflower growth after wet periods. The trail across the bajada and up into the mouth of the canyon is mostly flat, gaining only 300 feet over 3 miles. Most of that gain is at the very end as you approach the dam and edge along a narrow trail atop rock retaining wall. Sounds fun, eh? Hike early, bring plenty of water and a snack and watch for rattlers during the cooler parts of the day.

MILEAGE LOG

0.0 After making sure that you have a good supply of water, BEGIN near Area #9 on Ford Canyon Road. See the map. Cross Willow Canyon Wash and quickly join Ford Canyon Trail. Go LEFT and follow along above the wash.

0.5 PASS a spur trail to campground on right. CONTINUE as main trail leads north across an outwash plain, tops a small pass, descends and heads for Ford Canyon.

2.0 Trail get steeper and narrower as it enters the canyon and continues up toward the old abandoned rock dam.

3.0 Dam! Trail heads for serious back country. This is a good spot to eat lunch and TURNAROUND.

6.0 Back to Area #9 Trailhead.

DIRECTIONS: From downtown Phoenix take I-10 west for 20 miles to Cotton Lane Exit #124. Take a RIGHT and Head NORTH 7 miles on Cotton to Olive Avenue and turn LEFT. Go another 5 miles to the park entrance. Pick up a great free park topo map and CONTINUE 2.8 miles to Ford Canyon Road. Go LEFT another 0.7 miles to the trailhead at Area 9.

FORD CANYON TRAIL
WHITE TANKS

WHITE TANK MOUNTAINS
FORD CANYON TRAIL/ WILLOW SPRING LOOP

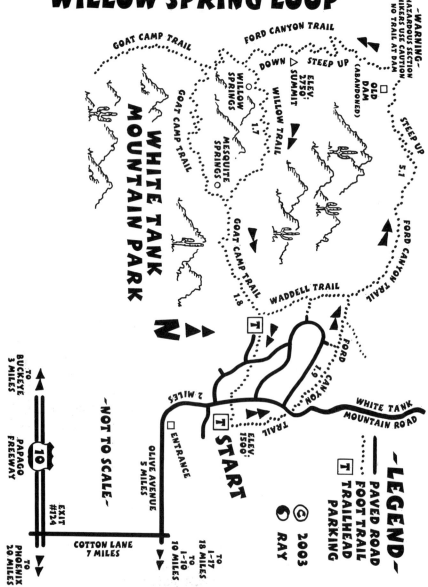

~WARNING~
HAZARDOUS SECTION
HIKERS USE CAUTION
NO TRAIL AT DAM

GOAT CAMP TRAIL

FORD CANYON TRAIL

DOWN ▷ STEEP UP

ELEV: 2750' SUMMIT

OLD DAM (ABANDONED)

STEEP UP 5.1

WILLOW SPRINGS

WILLOW TRAIL

1.7

MESQUITE SPRINGS

WHITE TANK MOUNTAIN PARK

GOAT CAMP TRAIL

FORD CANYON TRAIL

GOAT CAMP TRAIL 1.8

WADDELL TRAIL

T

N

FORD CANYON 1.9

WHITE TANK MOUNTAIN ROAD

2 MILES

ELEV: 1500'

TRAIL

START

T

□ ENTRANCE

OLIVE AVENUE 5 MILES

~NOT TO SCALE~

TO BUCKEYE 3 MILES

PAPAGO FREEWAY

10

EXIT #124

TO PHOENIX 20 MILES

COTTON LANE 7 MILES

TO I-17 18 MILES

TO I-10 10 MILES

~LEGEND~
PAVED ROAD
FOOT TRAIL
T TRAILHEAD PARKING
© 2003
RAY

WHITE TANK MOUNTAINS
FORD CANYON / WILLOW SPRING LOOP

DISTANCE: 10.5 MILES
TIME: ALL DAY
EFFORT: NO MERCY
TYPE: VERY LONG LOOP
ROUTE SKILL: MODERATE
(SIGNED, BUT SOME SKILL REQUIRED)
BEST SEASON: OCT to MAY
(NEVER IN SUMMER)
MAPS: PARK MAP
(GREAT FREE TOPO WHEN YOU ENTER)

AT-A-GLANCE

2900
ELEV. (FT.)
1400

0   **LOOP MILES**   10.5

PETS: NOT A GOOD IDEA
(VERY ROUGH & ROCKY TERRAIN)

DESCRIPTION: A serious challenge. You are not far from paved roads, but you visit some of the most scenic, rugged, remote back country in The Southwest. No water is available on the trail. Junctions are signed, but some hikers wander off trail and get lost, so pay attention. You must be in very fit condition. Do not bite off more than you can chew. Be ready for anything. Don't hike alone. Wear a hat, carry a compass, food and lots of water. Wear comfortable, tough shoes. The FREE park topo given when you enter comes in very handy.

MILEAGE LOG

0.0 START at FORD CANYON TRAILHEAD. See map. Cross White Tank Mountain Road and CONTINUE all around the trailhead staging areas to Waddell Trail Junction.

1.9 WADDELL TRAIL JUNCTION. Go RIGHT and CONTINUE.

3.9 OLD ABANDONED DAM. Trail gets rough. No distinct trail at dam. Find your way and CONTINUE. Begin STEEP CLIMB up Ford Canyon Trail to SUMMIT and then down.

7.0 JUNCTION with WILLOW TRAIL. Go LEFT to Springs.

7.2 WILLOW SPRINGS. Soak hot feet in cool water. AHHHH!

8.7 JUNCTION with GOAT CAMP TRAIL. Go LEFT. CONTINUE on Goat Camp Trail all the way back to the START.

10.5 Whew! Tough hike. You are The Cosmic Stud-muffin.

DIRECTIONS: From Phoenix take I-10 west 20 miles to Cotton Lane Exit #124. Go RIGHT and NORTH 7 miles on Cotton to Olive Avenue and turn LEFT. Go another 5 miles to park entrance. Continue 2 miles to Ford Canyon Trailhead on your RIGHT. Be absolutely sure to pick up the superb FREE park topo map at the park entrance before you begin.

WHITE TANK MOUNTAINS
WATERFALL TRAIL

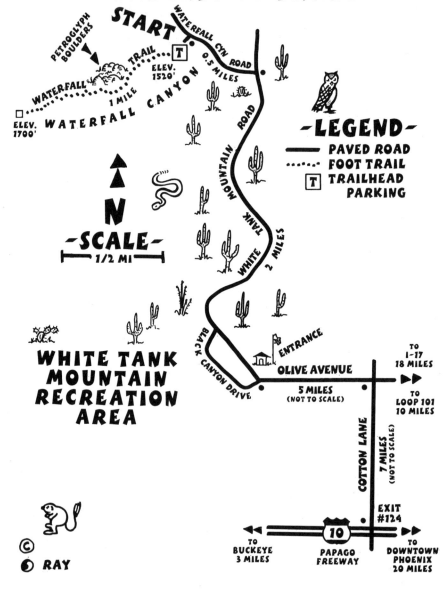

START

WATERFALL CYN ROAD
0.5 MILES

PETROGLYPH BOULDERS

WATERFALL TRAIL
T ELEV. 1520'

ELEV. 1700'

1 MILE

WATERFALL CANYON

MOUNTAIN ROAD

WHITE TANK

2 MILES

N

SCALE
1/2 MI

-LEGEND-
—— PAVED ROAD
······ FOOT TRAIL
T TRAILHEAD PARKING

WHITE TANK
MOUNTAIN
RECREATION
AREA

BLACK CANYON DRIVE

ENTRANCE

OLIVE AVENUE
5 MILES
(NOT TO SCALE)

TO
I-17
18 MILES

TO
LOOP 101
10 MILES

COTTON LANE

7 MILES
(NOT TO SCALE)

EXIT
#124

TO
BUCKEYE
3 MILES

10
PAPAGO
FREEWAY

TO
DOWNTOWN
PHOENIX
20 MILES

© RAY

WHITE TANK MOUNTAINS
WATERFALL TRAIL / PETROGLYPH PLAZA

DISTANCE: 2 MILES TOTAL
TIME: 1 to 2 HOURS
EFFORT: EASY AT FIRST
(GETS TOUGHER AT THE VERY END)
TYPE: OUT & BACK
ROUTE SKILL: EASY
BEST SEASON: OCT to MAY
WILDFLOWERS: FEB to APR
(PEAK SEASON MARCH)

AT-A-GLANCE

2500

ELEV. (FT.)

2000

0 **1-WAY MILES** 1.0

PETS: DOGS ON LEASH

DESCRIPTION: This short hike combines the best of what Phoenix has for us outdoorsy types. You find a palette of wildflowers, cacti galore, a cool canyon and hundreds of geometric designs drawn by Hohokam ancients over 1,000 years ago. The easy first half of the trail goes to the petroglyphs and is smooth enough for an outdoor enthusiast in a wheelchair. Bring some water and a leash for the dawg.

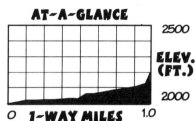

FAVORITE TRAIL
WORTH A JOURNEY

The shady, cool nature of Waterfall Canyon makes this a primo hike anytime, especially just after a rainy winter or summer monsoon. The canyon and waterfall are normally dry, but when water fills the pools at its base, you easily see why the Hohokam spent time here resting and carving designs in the thin dark desert varnish layer covering the light gray of these boulders. Hohokam hunted game and gathered plants around the base of these rugged vaulted granite peaks. Art was an expression of a desire to show their surroundings or a way to illustrate their prayers.

Waterfall Trail begins easy. At mile 0.4 you encounter the petroglyphs and benches for viewing. Then the way gets tough and rough as the canyon closes in. At mile 0.8, you find an old bullet riddled livestock tank. Finally, the bouldery trail reaches a gravelly dead end at mile 1.0. From here it's a short, risky hop up to the pools at the base of the falls. Careful!

DIRECTIONS: From downtown Phoenix take I-10 west for 20 miles to Cotton Lane Exit #124. Take a RIGHT and Head NORTH 7 miles on Cotton to Olive Avenue and turn LEFT. Go another 5 miles to park entrance. Pick up the great free park map and CONTINUE 2 miles to Waterfall Canyon Road. Go LEFT another 0.5 miles to the trailhead on your left.

WATERFALL TRAIL
WHITE TANKS

WHITE TANK MOUNTAINS
WILLOW TRAIL TO SPRINGS

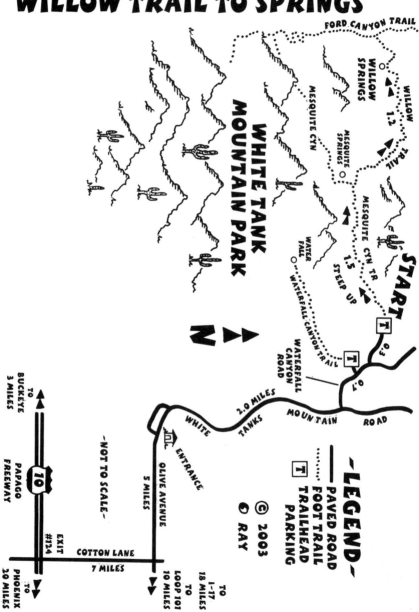

FORD CANYON TRAIL

WILLOW SPRINGS

WILLOW TRAIL 1.2

MESQUITE CYN

MESQUITE SPRINGS

WHITE TANK MOUNTAIN PARK

MESQUITE CYN TR 1.5

STEEP UP

WATER FALL

WATERFALL CANYON TRAIL

START

0.3

0.7

WATERFALL CANYON ROAD

N

2.0 MILES

WHITE TANKS MOUNTAIN ROAD

ENTRANCE

OLIVE AVENUE
5 MILES

COTTON LANE
7 MILES

TO BUCKEYE 3 MILES

PAPAGO FREEWAY

10

EXIT #124

TO PHOENIX 20 MILES

TO I-17 18 MILES

TO LOOP 101 10 MILES

—NOT TO SCALE—

—LEGEND—
- —— PAVED ROAD
- ⋯⋯ FOOT TRAIL
- T TRAILHEAD
- P PARKING

© 2003

☉ RAY

WHITE TANK MOUNTAINS
WILLOW SPRINGS

DISTANCE: 5.4 MILES TOTAL
TIME: 3 TO 4 HOURS
EFFORT: MODERATE
(FIRST MILE VERY STEEP, THEN EASY)
TYPE: OUT AND BACK
ROUTE SKILL: EASY
(SIGNED ALL THE WAY)
BEST SEASON: OCT to MAY
(DEEP CANYONS SHADY IN AFTERNOON)
WILDFLOWERS: FEB to APR

AT-A-GLANCE

2500

ELEV. (FT.)

1500

0   **1-WAY MILES**

PETS: DOGS ON LEASH

DESCRIPTION: The eastern slope of the White Tank Mountains outline the sky west of Phoenix. Composed of huge blocks of faulted white granite, eons of erosion have cut deep canyons into the mountains' flanks. Sudden, heavy seasonal rains create occasional waterfalls, pools called tanks and infrequent springs. One such verdant oasis in an otherwise steep, dry and forbidding landscape is Willow Springs, a pool surrounded by willows and steep mossy cliff walls offering shade from the otherwise relentless afternoon sun.

This popular hike is not extremely long, but starts off very steep and tough over the first mile or so, then mellows out making for an easy hike the rest of the way. Do not count on the springs for drinking water.

MILEAGE LOG

0.0 START steep climb from the trailhead. See map.
1.5 Trail splits. Best to go RIGHT. Left goes to quick visit to Mesquite Springs, but then continues out Mesquite Canyon Trail for a very long, epic walk home. GO RIGHT.
2.7 WILLOW SPRINGS. Inviting dog water. Good for a foot bath, but I don't suggest you (or your dog) take a sip. After a good sit-down go back the way you came.
5.4 Back to GO.

DIRECTIONS: From Phoenix take I-10 west 20 miles to Cotton Lane EXIT #124. Take a RIGHT and Head NORTH for 7 miles on Cotton to Olive Avenue and turn LEFT. Go another 5 miles to park entrance. Continue 2 miles to Waterfall Canyon Road. Go LEFT about a mile to Ramada Road and go LEFT again to the trailhead at the end of Ramada Road. Be sure to Pick up a new really good FREE topo park map now available when you enter. Very helpful.

SAN FRANCISCO PEAKS
HUMPHREYS PEAK TRAIL

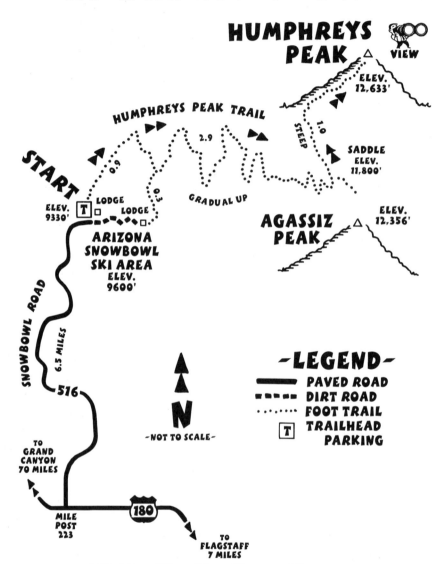

HUMPHREYS
PEAK △ 👀 VIEW

ELEV.
12,633'

HUMPHREYS PEAK TRAIL

2.9

STEEP

1.0

0.9

0.3

SADDLE
ELEV.
11,800'

START

GRADUAL UP

ELEV.
9330'

T LODGE
LODGE

ELEV.
12,356'

AGASSIZ
PEAK △

ARIZONA
SNOWBOWL
SKI AREA
ELEV.
9600'

SNOWBOWL ROAD

6.5 MILES

516

N
—NOT TO SCALE—

—LEGEND—

▬▬▬▬▬	PAVED ROAD
▬ ▬ ▬ ▬	DIRT ROAD
··········	FOOT TRAIL
T	TRAILHEAD PARKING

TO
GRAND
CANYON
70 MILES

MILE
POST
223

🛡180

TO
FLAGSTAFF
7 MILES

FLAGSTAFF © RAY

HIGH COUNTRY
FLAGSTAFF: HUMPHREY'S PEAK TRAIL

DISTANCE: 9.6 MILES
TIME: 4-6 HOURS
EFFORT: IT'S TOUGH
TYPE: UP AND BACK DOWN
ROUTE SKILL: EASY
(WELL SIGNED)
BEST SEASON: JUN TO OCT
(SNOW IN WINTER)
PETS: DOGS ON LEASH

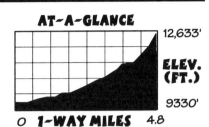

AT-A-GLANCE

12,633'

ELEV.
(FT.)

9330'

O **1-WAY MILES** 4.8

DESCRIPTION: Excellent for those wicked hot summer days when the Phoenix mercury climbs up, up, up and then off the scale. On just such a day you may get higher than a proverbial hippie in a helicopter. You will stand above all others in The Land of AZ . . . ruler of all you survey. Well, let's not get too carried away, but you will ascend to the top of Humphreys Peak, highest of the San Francisco Peaks and highest point in Arizona at 12,633 ft. It's up there!

Plan for an all day outing. Bring food and water as well as protective clothing. If it begins to cloud up, it is time to bail. You would not be the first nor the last to be blown to kingdom come by a lightning bolt at this elevation. Talk about your bad hair day!

Have a look at the map. Beginning from the Snowbowl lodge parking area, you cross an open grassy meadow then climb up through a dark, dense forest of conifer and aspen to a trail junction. Continue LEFT all the way up to timber-line at 10,500 ft. A barren rocky saddle is ahead just above at 11,800 ft. Once in the saddle the trail splits. You bear LEFT and continue up, up, up over a series of three heart breaking false summits over the final mile until you finally peak out at 12,633 ft. and a stupendous 360° view.

For the respiratorily challenged, Arizona Snowbowl offers a summer chairlift skyride up neighboring Agassiz Peak for a great view to the north, south and west from an observation platform.

DIRECTIONS: North out of Flag 7 miles on Highway 180 to milepost 223. Go right onto Snow Bowl Road for 6.5 miles then turn left to the end of the parking area just below the lodge. Good spot for apres hike brews and snackage!

FLAGSTAFF: PEAK TRAIL
HIGH COUNTRY

RED MOUNTAIN

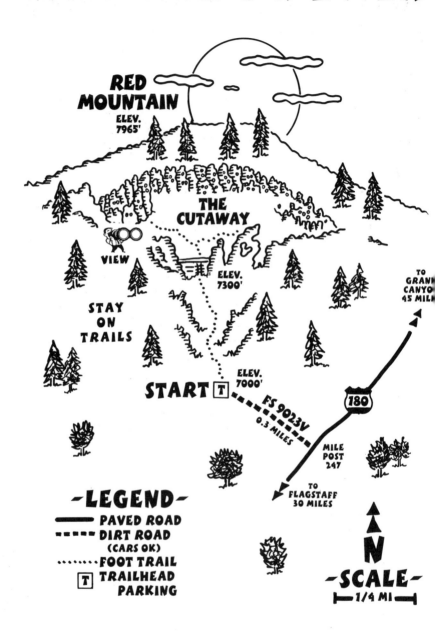

RED
MOUNTAIN
ELEV.
7965'

THE
CUTAWAY

VIEW

ELEV.
7300'

STAY
ON
TRAILS

START T ELEV.
7000'

FS 9023V
0.3 MILES

180

TO
GRAND
CANYON
45 MILES

MILE
POST
247

TO
FLAGSTAFF
30 MILES

-LEGEND-
———— PAVED ROAD
----- DIRT ROAD
(CARS OK)
·········· FOOT TRAIL
T TRAILHEAD
PARKING

N
-SCALE-
├── 1/4 MI ──┤

FLAGSTAFF

HIGH COUNTRY
FLAGSTAFF: *RED MOUNTAIN*

DISTANCE: 2.6 MILES TOTAL
TIME: 2 HOURS
EFFORT: DANG EASY
TYPE: OUT AND BACK
ROUTE SKILL: SIGNED
BEST SEASON: ALL YEAR
(SNOW POSSIBLE IN WINTER)
PETS: BRING A LEASH

AT-A-GLANCE

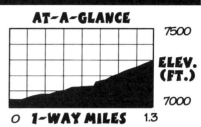

7500

ELEV. (FT.)

7000

0   **1-WAY MILES**   1.3

DESCRIPTION: Easy hike to *inside* a mountian. Red Mountain is like other small mountains or volcanic cinder hills that dot this cool high country area north of The San Francisco Peaks *except* its eastern face has collapsed and fallen away revealing a cutaway core.

Bring binoculars. If I were a bird, I'd live here! The exposed cliffs of *The Cutaway* are covered with *juecos* or big swiss cheese holes caused by gas bubbles as the mountain was formed making for hundreds of bird condos. Weather sculpted hoodoos and goblins with eye holes look for all the world like a chorus of Mr. Potato Heads keeping their eyes on you. Redrock flutes, slots and butt cracks are every-where on the eroded cliff face. Summer mornings are best for viewing and photos of this mondo bizarro scene.

The easy, well marked trail heads up an old road then into a wash at 0.8 miles and continues. At 1.2 miles you meet a 7 ft. high rock dam blocking *The Gateway*. Up and over the ladder or go up the nearby steep cinder path. Continue just a few more feet and you're there. Explore, but use caution. The surfaces of this steep scenery are NOT suitable for climbing and may flake off in your hand. Stay on trails or slickrock. Footprints may begin new avenues for erosion leaving ugly scars.

DIRECTIONS: From Phoenix go NORTH on I-17 to Flagstaff. The 130 mile drive should take about 2 hours. Have a snack then head North out of Flagstaff on Highway 180 toward Grand Canyon for another 30 miles to milepost 247. Follow map to the parking area.

"If you don't know where you're going, any road will do."
-George Harrison

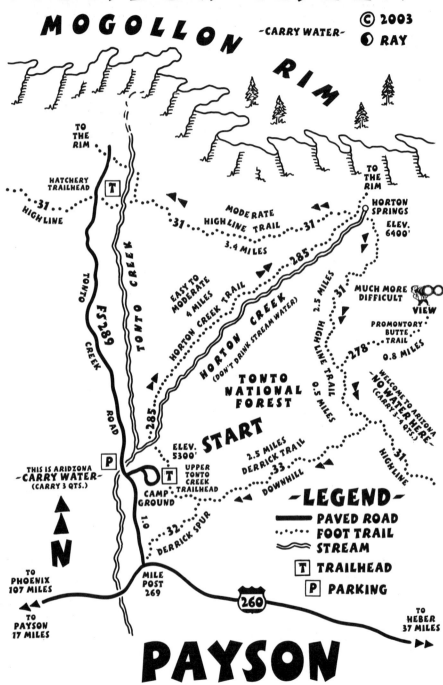

HORTON CREEK

MOGOLLON RIM

-CARRY WATER-

© 2003
RAY

TO THE RIM

HATCHERY TRAILHEAD

31 HIGH LINE

TONTO CREEK

FS 289

T

MODERATE HIGH LINE TRAIL
3.4 MILES

31

31

285

TO THE RIM

HORTON SPRINGS
ELEV. 6400'

MUCH MORE DIFFICULT

VIEW

EASY TO MODERATE 4 MILES

HORTON CREEK TRAIL

285

HORTON CREEK
(DON'T DRINK STREAM WATER)

31

2.5 MILES

HIGH LINE TRAIL

0.5 MILES

PROMONTORY BUTTE TRAIL
0.8 MILES

278

~WELCOME TO ARIZONA~
NO WATER HERE
(CARRY 3-4 QTS.)

31 HIGHLINE

CREEK

ROAD

TONTO NATIONAL FOREST

START

ELEV. 5300'

2.5 MILES
DERRICK TRAIL

33

DOWNHILL

THIS IS ARIDZONA
-CARRY WATER-
(CARRY 3 QTS.)

P

UPPER TONTO CREEK TRAILHEAD

T

CAMP GROUND

N

1.0

32

DERRICK SPUR

-LEGEND-

PAVED ROAD
FOOT TRAIL
STREAM
T TRAILHEAD
P PARKING

TO PHOENIX 107 MILES

TO PAYSON 17 MILES

MILE POST 269

260

TO HEBER 37 MILES

PAYSON

DISTANCE: 2 TO 9.5 MILES
TIME: 2 TO 6 HOURS
EFFORT: EASY TO MEDIUM
(LONG LOOP RATED DIFFICULT)
TYPE: OUT AND BACK
ROUTE SKILL: EASY
(FOLLOW THE CREEK)
BEST SEASON: APR TO NOV
(WARM SUMMERS, SNOWY WINTERS)
PETS: CARRY A LEASH

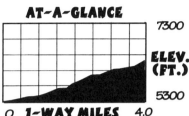

AT-A-GLANCE

7300

**ELEV.
(FT.)**

5300

0　**1-WAY MILES**　4.0
HORTON CREEK TRAIL

DESCRIPTION: While still darn warm in summer, never the less a huge respite from the searing Phoenix oven, HORTON CREEK TRAIL runs a path along and in-and-out of splashing Horton Creek. Stroll up an easy old road above the creek or a moderate path right down by the stream. Enjoy the sight of small waterfalls and maybe a trout or two. I was happy in my Tevas getting my feet in the creek every opportunity. As a classic leafy FALL COLOR HIKE, the 1000' climb spread over 4 miles is not hard. You can go far as you like and turn around or go all the way to gushing Horton Spring for the 8 mile turn-and-burn.

   If you are more hard core and adventurous, you can make a 9.5 mile loop by turning RIGHT at Horton Spring and retun via a short section of the infamous 50 mile Highline Trail PLUS 2.5 miles down thru aligator juniper on DERRICK TRAIL. It's simple. See the map. This 3 mile stretch of the Highline is rough and steep with some big ups and downs. At 9.5 miles total, this loop will not be much longer than the simple out and back to the spring, but much tougher. No water here.

   And then then a severe version for those with reason open to question . . . look at the map. PROMINTORY BUTTE TRAIL (short, steep and brushy) is a 0.8 mile spur off Highline to a mesa and a view. Worth it only to us few insane-os.

DIRECTIONS: From Phoenix go 90 miles NORTHEAST on Beeline HWY 87 to Payson. In Payson, turn RIGHT (EAST) on HWY 260 another 17 miles to milepost 269 and turn LEFT onto Tonto Creek Road, FS 289. Go 1 more mile, cross the bridge and park in the picnic area. The trailhead is back across the bridge in the campground.

"To find the flow, you must first lose reason."
-The Buddha

PAYSON: HORTON CREEK **HIGH COUNTRY**

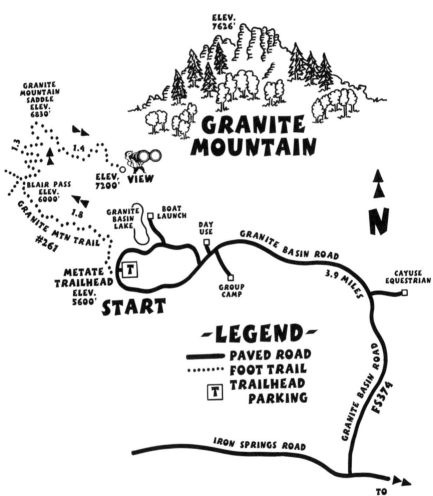

GRANITE MOUNTAIN VISTA © 2003 ⊙ RAY

ELEV. 7626'

GRANITE MOUNTAIN

GRANITE MOUNTAIN SADDLE ELEV. 6830'

1.3

1.4

BLAIR PASS ELEV. 6000'

ELEV. 7200' VIEW

1.8

GRANITE MTN TRAIL #261

GRANITE BASIN LAKE

BOAT LAUNCH

DAY USE

GRANITE BASIN ROAD

N

METATE TRAILHEAD ELEV. 5600'

T

START

GROUP CAMP

3.9 MILES

CAYUSE EQUESTRIAN

GRANITE BASIN ROAD

FS374

~LEGEND~
— PAVED ROAD
...... FOOT TRAIL
T TRAILHEAD PARKING

IRON SPRINGS ROAD

TO PRESCOTT COURTHOUSE SQUARE VIA MONTEZUMA/WHIPPLE/ IRON SPRINGS ROAD 4.7 MILES

PRESCOTT

HIGH COUNTRY
PRESCOTT: *GRANITE MOUNTAIN VISTA*

DISTANCE: 9 MILES TOTAL
TIME: 5 TO 6 HOURS
EFFORT: MEDIUM
(CLIMBS MODERATED BY SWITCHBACKS)
TYPE: OUT AND BACK
ROUTE SKILL: SIGNED
BEST SEASON: ALL YEAR
(SOUTH FACING, VERY WARM IN SUMMER)
PETS: BRING A LEASH

AT-A-GLANCE

8000

ELEV. (FT.)

5500

0   **1-WAY MILES**   4.5

DESCRIPTION: "Nature's whims oft times can produce such grotesque and ponderous jumbles of massive rock material that man must stand in fascinated awe and admiration." That unknown 19th century author hit the nail right on the head. Boulders and battlements, spires and buttes, hoodoos and goblins . . . all carved by nature out of pink Precambrian granite over a span of 2 billion years. Thumb Butte, Granite Dells and Granite Mountain are all typical of this process.

The soaring cliffs are ideal nesting habitat for peregrine falcons. Pinyon, juniper, manzanita, aspen and ponderosa pine carpet the wilderness around the mountain. The panorama includes the summit of Granite Mountain and Granite Basin Lake nearby; Prescott, Thumb Butte and Granite Dells to the east and The Bradshaws in the distance. Although cooler than Phoenix, Granite Mountain is quite warm in summer. Start early. Carry plenty of water.

MILEAGE LOG

0.0   BEGIN Metate Trailhead. See the map. Granite Mountain Trail #261 climbs 400' in the first 1.8 miles.

1.8   Blair Pass. 3-way JUNCTION. Go RIGHT and UP gradual switchbacks to Granite Mountain Saddle.

3.1   SADDLE. Good views of Granite Mountain's face. The trail levels off and continues to Granite Mountain Vista.

4.5   VISTA. Soak up the view and return the way you came.

DIRECTIONS: From Phoenix go 60 miles NORTH on I-17 to Cordes Junction Exit #262 then follow signs and HWY 69 another 33 miles to Courthouse Square in Prescott. Take Montezuma Street NORTH, which becomes Whipple which becomes Iron Springs Road. You're nearly there. Now look at the map. There is a small fee to park at the trailhead.

PRESCOTT: GRANITE MOUNTAIN
HIGH COUNTRY

WEST FORK OF OAK CREEK

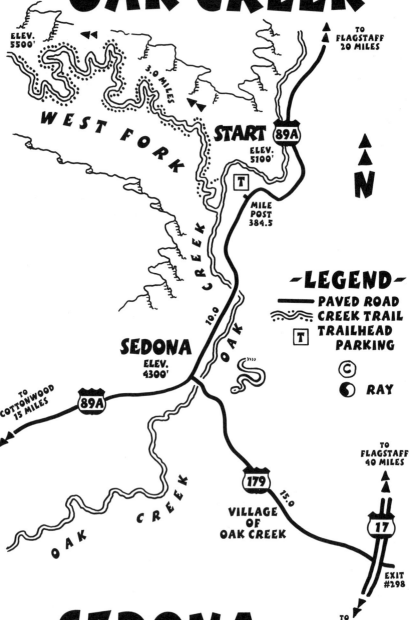

ELEV. 5500'

3.0 MILES

WEST FORK

START
89A
ELEV. 5100'

T

MILE POST 384.5

TO FLAGSTAFF 20 MILES

N

-LEGEND-
—— PAVED ROAD
〰️ CREEK TRAIL
T TRAILHEAD PARKING
Ⓒ RAY

OAK CREEK

SEDONA
ELEV. 4300'

TO COTTONWOOD 15 MILES
89A

179
15.0

VILLAGE OF OAK CREEK

OAK CREEK

TO FLAGSTAFF 40 MILES

17

EXIT #298

TO PHOENIX 90 MILES

SEDONA

HIGH COUNTRY
SEDONA: WEST FORK OF OAK CREEK

DISTANCE: 3 to 6 MILES
TIME: 2-3 HOURS
EFFORT: FAIRLY EASY
TYPE: OUT AND BACK
ROUTE SKILL: EASY
(FOLLOW THE CREEK)
BEST SEASON: APR to NOV
(SNOW IN WINTER)
PETS: DOGS ON LEASH

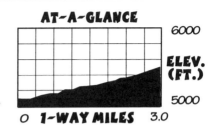

AT-A-GLANCE

6000

ELEV.
(FT.)

5000

O **1-WAY MILES** 3.0

DESCRIPTION: Perfect almost anytime, but especially when Phoenix fires up the summer oven. Sedona's West Fork of Oak Creek is 2.5 hours away and 3,500 feet higher. The idyllic little stream that is a fork of Oak Creek snakes down out of Secret Mountain Wilderness through sculpted redrock Coconino sandstone canyon cliffs 1000 ft. high.

Summer is great. Subtract 25° from Phoenix high temps. In spring, songbirds trill and dot trees with flashes of color. Fall is magic time. Red and gold pastels of maple and oak leaves drift like tiny boats along mirrored pools connected by a softly splashing brook. No wonder West Fork is the most visited trail in Coconino National Forest.

The marked path wanders three easy miles upstream under views of towering terra cotta cliffs. Wear tennies or Tevas as West Fork Trail zig-zags across the shallow creek on stepping stones and quick splashes in shallow water. However, if you continue way upstream for more of the creek's entire 14 mile length to where it begins near Woody Mountain Road west of Flagstaff, be ready for lots of stream bed wading, boulder hopping and swimming.

DIRECTIONS: Head NORTH out of Phoenix for 90 miles on I-17 toward Flagstaff. Take Sedona Exit #298 and go LEFT (NORTH) 15 miles on HWY 179 through Village of Oak Creek and on to Sedona. Turn RIGHT (NORTH) onto HWY 89A at the "Y" intersection in Sedona. CONTINUE on HWY 89A another 10 miles to milepost 384.5 and into the West Fork Trailhead fee parking area. There are bathrooms at the trailhead and a $5 fee to park.

SEDONA: WEST FORK TRAIL
HIGH COUNTRY

"It ain't what we know that causes problems.
It's what we know that just ain't so."

WET BEAVER CREEK
CREEK
BELL TRAIL

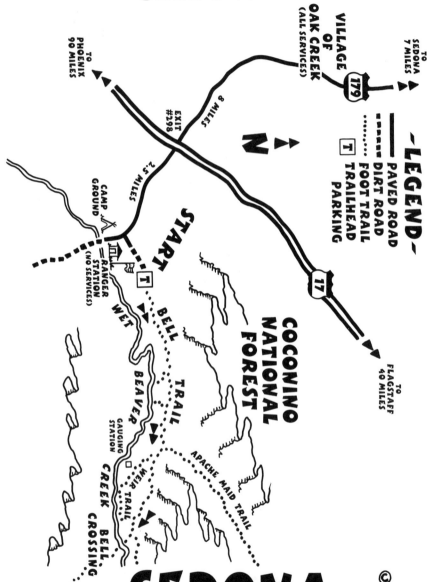

TO SEDONA 7 MILES

VILLAGE OF OAK CREEK (ALL SERVICES)

179

TO PHOENIX 90 MILES

EXIT #298

8 MILES

N

17

TO FLAGSTAFF 40 MILES

-LEGEND-
PAVED ROAD
DIRT ROAD
FOOT TRAIL
T TRAILHEAD PARKING

2.5 MILES

CAMP GROUND

START

T

RANGER STATION (NO SERVICES)

WET

BEAVER

BELL

TRAIL

GAUGING STATION

WEIR TRAIL

APACHE MAID TRAIL

COCONINO NATIONAL FOREST

CREEK

BELL CROSSING

SEDONA

© RAY

DISTANCE: 8 MILES
TIME: 3-4 HOURS
EFFORT: MODERATE
TYPE: OUT AND BACK
ROUTE SKILL: EASY
(SIGNED/FOLLOW THE CREEK)
BEST SEASON: ALL YEAR
(VERY WARM IN SUMMER)
PETS: BRING A LEASH

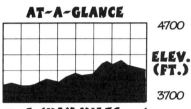

AT-A-GLANCE

4700

ELEV. (FT.)

3700

O **1-WAY MILES** 4

DESCRIPTION: Water running clear and clean with deep pools and redrock cliffs for diving sounds like just the ticket when that Arizona sun gets cranking hot. There is a fairly easy trail to just such a magic spot at Bell's Crossing with spurs along the way to access and enjoy Wet Beaver Creek just south of Sedona.

Bell Trail was built by Charlie Bell in the 1930s to run his cattle up to summer pasture along the Mogollon Rim. Never did this lonesome cowboy envision so many hikers along his splashing creek. A bit crowded on weekends, but still pleasant.

As you leave the parking area, the trail is wide and smooth, but runs through private property. You must go about a quarter mile before you can drop down to the creek. Bell Trail continues easy rolling until you have gone about three miles. Then you go up and over high above the creek. Finally, Bell Trail drops down to Beaver Creek at the cliffs, ledges and pools of Bell's Crossing. Always use caution when diving. Look before you leap.

There are no public services at the ranger station. You'll find a formal campground near the ranger station and there are a few wilderness creekside spots just below the gauging station off the Weir Trail. See the map.

DIRECTIONS: Paved all the way to the trailhead, Bell Trail and Wet Beaver Creek are 90 miles NORTH of Phoenix just off I-17 and very easy to find. Take EXIT #298 where I-17 meets HWY 179 about 15 miles south of Sedona. Follow the signs to the parking area about 2 miles EAST.

"Beware of enterprises that require new clothes."
- Henry David Thoreau

SEDONA:WET BEAVER CREEK
HIGH COUNTRY

~ BACK WORD ~

Hi, I'm Cosmic Ray and despite the name I am a real person. In towns all over the great state of Arizona folks are often applied a handle or nickname to distinguish them from others of the same name. No kidding, I was really given this name by friends and it stuck. Why Cosmic? Why not. Good as any, I reckon.

My cartoony maps are adapted from my GPS work, topos and forest service charts as well as city, county and state maps. They are oriented north and as close to scale as I can make them and still fit on a page. I like to think they have a human look rather than being drawn by a computer. I've been told they look more like notes from a buddy than a handbook. I like that because it's true. I hope you have as much fun with this guide as I had creating it.

Humble thanks to my many fine friends who helped with ideas, advice and sweat. A special thank you to my very talented young pal Ben Proctor for his cartoon art. More thanks to wife Marcia and *Cosmic Grommet* Elena Marie who add love and understanding. With friends and family, we can wander forever and never be lost. Wherever you go, there you are!

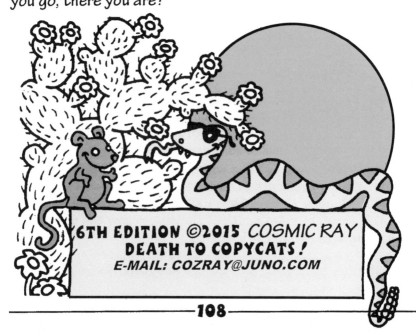

6TH EDITION ©2015 *COSMIC RAY*
DEATH TO COPYCATS!
E-MAIL: COZRAY@JUNO.COM

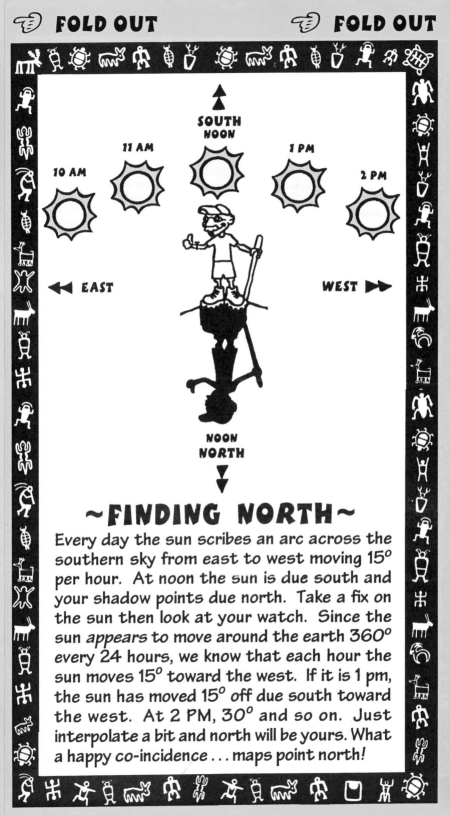

**SOUTH
NOON**

11 AM

10 AM

1 PM

2 PM

◄◄ EAST

WEST ►►

NOON
NORTH

~FINDING NORTH~

Every day the sun scribes an arc across the southern sky from east to west moving 15° per hour. At noon the sun is due south and your shadow points due north. Take a fix on the sun then look at your watch. Since the sun *appears* to move around the earth 360° every 24 hours, we know that each hour the sun moves 15° toward the west. If it is 1 pm, the sun has moved 15° off due south toward the west. At 2 PM, 30° and so on. Just interpolate a bit and north will be yours. What a happy co-incidence . . . maps point north!

~THE WEATHER~

	JAN	FEB	MAR	APR	MAY	JUN	JUL	AUG	SEP	OCT	NOV	DEC
AVERAGE HIGH TEMPERATURE (°F)	66	70	75	84	93	103	105	103	99	88	75	66
AVERAGE LOW TEMPERATURE (°F)	41	44	49	55	64	72	80	79	72	61	48	42
HIGHEST RECORDED TEMPERATURE (°F)	88	92	100	105	113	122	121	116	118	107	93	88
LOWEST RECORDED TEMPERATURE (°F)	17	22	25	37	40	51	66	61	47	34	27	22
AVERAGE PRECIPITATION (INCHES)	0.8	0.6	0.9	0.3	0.1	0.1	0.8	1.0	0.7	0.6	0.6	0.9
AVERAGE POSSIBILITY OF SUNSHINE	78%	80%	84%	89%	93%	94%	85%	85%	89%	88%	84%	78%